2020-2021 HESI Live Review Workbook for the

NCLEX-RN® EXAM, Revised Reprint

E. Tina Cuellar, PhD, RN
Director, HESI Live Review
Elsevier Reading Courses
Nursing and Health Professions
Houston, Texas

ELSEVIER

Elsevier
3251 Riverport Lane
St. Louis, MO 63043

2020–2021 HESI LIVE REVIEW WORKBOOK FOR THE NCLEX-RN® EXAM,
Revised Reprint   ISBN: 978-0-323-79690-3

Notices

Knowledge and best practice in this field are constantly changing. As new research and experience broaden our understanding, changes in research methods, professional practices, or medical treatment may become necessary.

Practitioners and researchers must always rely on their own experience and knowledge in evaluating and using any information, methods, compounds, or experiments described herein. In using such information or methods they should be mindful of their own safety and the safety of others, including parties for whom they have a professional responsibility.

With respect to any drug or pharmaceutical products identified, readers are advised to check the most current information provided (i) on procedures featured or (ii) by the manufacturer of each product to be administered, to verify the recommended dose or formula, the method and duration of administration, and contraindications. It is the responsibility of practitioners, relying on their own experience and knowledge of their patients, to make diagnoses, to determine dosages and the best treatment for each individual patient, and to take all appropriate safety precautions.

To the fullest extent of the law, neither the Publisher nor the authors, contributors, or editors, assume any liability for any injury and/or damage to persons or property as a matter of products liability, negligence or otherwise, or from any use or operation of any methods, products, instructions, or ideas contained in the material herein.

The Publisher NCLEX®, NCLEX-RN®, and NCLEX-PN® are registered trademarks of the National Council of State Boards of Nursing, Inc.

Director, Traditional Education Content: Tamara Myers
Senior Content Development Manager: Luke Held
Senior Content Development Specialist: Jennifer Wade
Publishing Services Manager: Shereen Jameel
Project Manager: Kamatchi Madhavan
Designer: Bridget Hoette

Printed in the United States of America

Last digit is the print number: 9 8 7 6 5 4

Contributors

Angela Gail Atwood, PhD, RN
Assistant Professor of Nursing
School of Nursing
Campbellsville University
Campbellsville, Kentucky

Joanna Cain, BSN, BA
President & Founder
Auctorial Pursuits, LLC
Boulder, Colorado

Marcia Clevesy, DNP, WHNP-BC
Assistant Professor
School of Nursing
University of Nevada, Las Vegas
Las Vegas, Nevada

Holly Johanna Diesel, PhD, MSN, BSN, BA
Nursing Department
Goldfarb School of Nursing at Barnes-Jewish College
St. Louis, Missouri

Amber Essman, DNP, MSN, FNP-BC
Ambulatory Care
Nationwide Children's Hospital
Columbus, Ohio

Helen Freeman, MSN, BSN, ADN
President
Keep It Simple for Success Nursing Education Consultant
Asheville, North Carolina

Virginia Jean Hallenbeck, BSN, MS, DNP
Visiting Professor
Nursing Department
Chamberlain School of Nursing
Downer's Grove, Illinois;
Adjunct Faculty
Nursing Department
Indiana Wesleyan University
Marian, Indiana

Sandra K. Jenkins, BSN, MS, MSN, PhD
Visiting Assistant Professor
Nursing Department
University of Houston Clear Lake
Houston, Texas

Necole Leland, DNP, MSN, RN, PNP, CPN
Assistant Professor
School of Nursing
University of Nevada
Las Vegas, Nevada

Linda Turchin, RN, MSN, CNE
Professor Emeritus
Nursing Department
Fairmont State University
Fairmont, West Virginia

Test-Taking Strategies and Study Guide

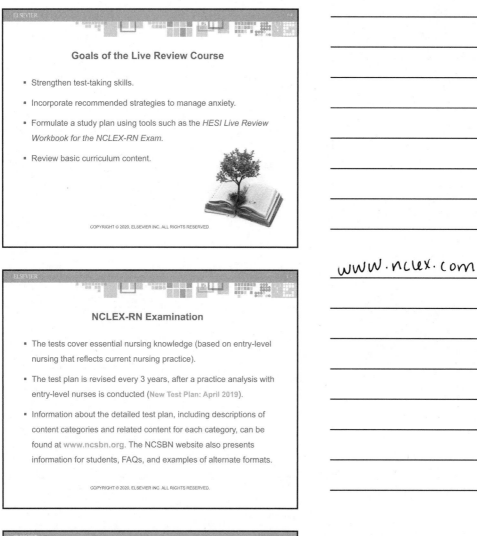

Goals of the Live Review Course

- Strengthen test-taking skills.
- Incorporate recommended strategies to manage anxiety.
- Formulate a study plan using tools such as the *HESI Live Review Workbook for the NCLEX-RN Exam.*
- Review basic curriculum content.

NCLEX-RN Examination

- The tests cover essential nursing knowledge (based on entry-level nursing that reflects current nursing practice).
- The test plan is revised every 3 years, after a practice analysis with entry-level nurses is conducted (New Test Plan: April 2019).
- Information about the detailed test plan, including descriptions of content categories and related content for each category, can be found at www.ncsbn.org. The NCSBN website also presents information for students, FAQs, and examples of alternate formats.

Organization of NCLEX-RN Test Plan: Client Need Categories

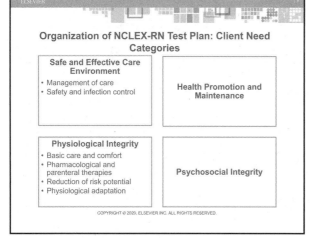

Safe and Effective Care Environment	Health Promotion and Maintenance
• Management of care • Safety and infection control	

Physiological Integrity	Psychosocial Integrity
• Basic care and comfort • Pharmacological and parenteral therapies • Reduction of risk potential • Physiological adaptation	

www.nclex.com

Organization of Test Plan: Integrated Processes

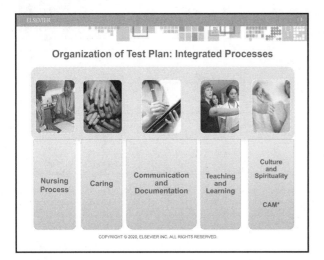

| Nursing Process | Caring | Communication and Documentation | Teaching and Learning | Culture and Spirituality CAM* |

Test Administration: Computerized Adaptive Testing

- Difficulty level is tailored to the candidate's ability.
- All candidates must answer a minimum of 75 items.
- The maximum number of items during the allotted ~~8~~-hour period is ~~265~~.

5   145

About Test Item Questions

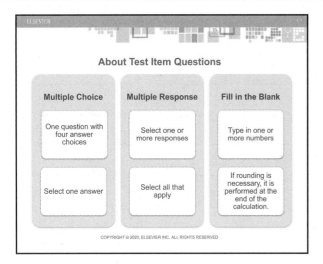

Multiple Choice	Multiple Response	Fill in the Blank
One question with four answer choices	Select one or more responses	Type in one or more numbers
Select one answer	Select all that apply	If rounding is necessary, it is performed at the end of the calculation.

*Med classifications

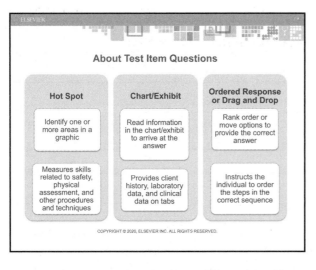

About Test Item Questions

Hot Spot	Chart/Exhibit	Ordered Response or Drag and Drop
Identify one or more areas in a graphic	Read information in the chart/exhibit to arrive at the answer	Rank order or move options to provide the correct answer
Measures skills related to safety, physical assessment, and other procedures and techniques	Provides client history, laboratory data, and clinical data on tabs	Instructs the individual to order the steps in the correct sequence

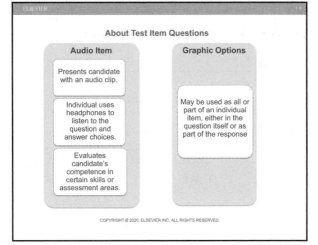

About Test Item Questions

Audio Item	Graphic Options
Presents candidate with an audio clip.	May be used as all or part of an individual item, either in the question itself or as part of the response
Individual uses headphones to listen to the question and answer choices.	
Evaluates candidate's competence in certain skills or assessment areas.	

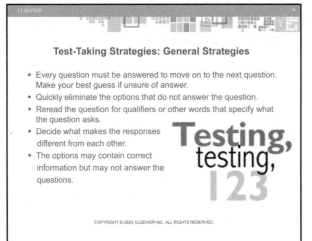

Test-Taking Strategies: General Strategies

- Every question must be answered to move on to the next question. Make your best guess if unsure of answer.
- Quickly eliminate the options that do not answer the question.
- Reread the question for qualifiers or other words that specify what the question asks.
- Decide what makes the responses different from each other.
- The options may contain correct information but may not answer the questions.

Testing, testing, 123

Test-Taking Strategies for Your Toolbox

•Use ABCs

- Clients with airway problems or interventions are top priority.
- Actual CPR = C-A-B
- Acute before chronic

hemodynamic Stability: BP
target min 100 > SBP

Test-Taking Strategies for Your Toolbox

Maslow's Hierarchy of Needs

- Address physiological needs first, followed by safety and security needs, love and belonging needs, self-esteem needs, and, finally, self-actualization needs.
- When a physiological need is not addressed in the question, look for the option that addresses safety.

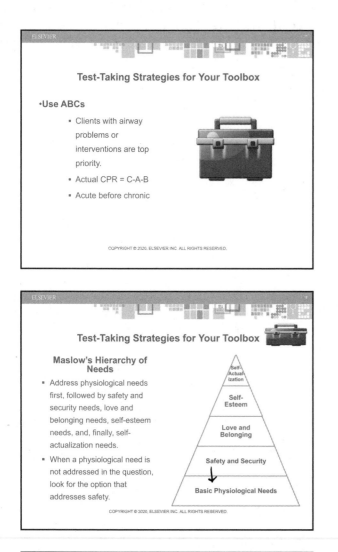

Self-Actualization
Self-Esteem
Love and Belonging
Safety and Security
Basic Physiological Needs

Are the physiological needs
met? Is the environment
safe?

Test-Taking Strategies for Your Toolbox

Carefully determine the steps of the nursing process.

Assessment requires gathering and verification of data.
Analysis requires interpreting data, communicating the diagnoses, and determining the health team's ability to meet needs.
Planning requires knowledge of prioritization and organization.
Implementation reflects delegation and assignment of tasks.
Evaluation compares actual outcomes with expected outcomes.

Do you have all assessment
info to intervene?

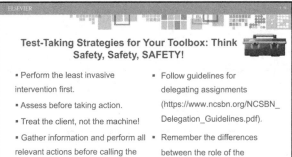

Test-Taking Strategies for Your Toolbox: Think Safety, Safety, SAFETY!

- Perform the least invasive intervention first.
- Assess before taking action.
- Treat the client, not the machine!
- Gather information and perform all relevant actions before calling the healthcare provider (HCP).
- Determine which client to assess first (most at risk, most physiologically unstable).

- Follow guidelines for delegating assignments (https://www.ncsbn.org/NCSBN_Delegation_Guidelines.pdf).
- Remember the differences between the role of the licensed nurse and the role of unlicensed assistive personnel (UAP).

More Test-Taking Strategies

Notifying the healthcare provider is a **red flag item**. Think about the appropriate nursing actions to take **prior** to notifying the HCP.

Common interventions include the following:
- Small, frequent feedings
- Recommended fluid intake: "3 L/day"
- Alternate rest with activity
- Conserve energy with any activity

Teaching Points

- Risk factors: modifiable versus nonmodifiable
- Prevention and wellness promotion
- New medications and self-care instructions
- Client empowerment
- Anticipatory guidance
- Incorporating client education information into lifestyle, culture, and spiritual beliefs

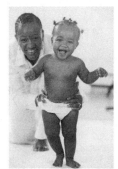

Clarification of Acronyms

Healthcare Provider (HCP)	Prescriptions	Unlicensed Assistive Personnel (UAP)
Physician/ Physician assistant	Orders written by licensed HCPs	Client care technician
Nurse practitioner		Nursing assistant
		Nurse's aide

Keep Memorization to a Minimum

- Growth and development milestones
- Crisis intervention
- Lab values
- Drug classifications
- Immunizations
- Stages of death and dying
- Principles of teaching/learning
- Stages of pregnancy and fetal growth
- Nurse Practice Act: Standards of Practice and Delegation

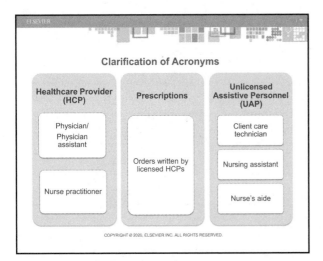

Don't FORGET!

Strategies for Success in Answering NCLEX-RN Questions: Essential Steps

1. Determine if the style of the question is

    + positive +
    or
    – negative –

2. Find the key words in the question.

3. Rephrase the question in your own words and answer the question.

4. Rule out options.

Is the Question in a Positive or Negative Style?

A *positive style* may ask what the nurse should do or the best or first action to implement.

A *negative style* may ask what the nurse should avoid, which prescription the nurse should question, or which behavior indicates the need for reteaching the client.

The Next Steps

Identify **key words** or phrases that provide the critical information.
- The age of the client, the setting, the timing, a set of symptoms or behaviors, diagnoses, medications, lab values, vital signs
- For example, the nursing actions for a 10-year-old, 1-day postoperative client are different from those for a 70-year-old, 1-hour postoperative client.

Rephrase the Question
- This helps eliminate nonessential information in the question and helps you determine the correct answer
- Ask yourself, "What is the question *really* asking?"
- Before looking at the choices, rephrase the question in your own words. Then answer the question.

Rule Out Options
- Based on your knowledge, identify any options that are clearly incorrect.
- Mentally mark through those options on the computer monitor.
- Differentiate among the remaining options, using prior knowledge of the subject and related nursing principles (e.g., roles of the nurse, nursing process, ABCs, Maslow's Hierarchy of Needs).

Appropriate Knowledge

- Use the appropriate knowledge to answer questions.
  - **Do not** respond based on:
    - *Your* past client care experiences or agency
    - A familiar phrase or term
    - "Of course, *I* would have already ..."
    - What *you* think is *realistic*
    - *Your* children, pregnancies, parents, elders, personal response to a drug, and so on
  - **Do** respond based on:
    - ABCs
    - Scientific, behavioral, sociological principles
    - Principles of teaching/learning
    - Maslow's Hierarchy of Needs
    - Nursing process
  - Answer based only on what the question asks—no more, no less.
    - NCLEX-RN ideal hospital
    - Basic anatomy and physiology
    - Critical thinking

Question

A client has not had a bowel movement in 2 days and reports this information to the nurse. Which intervention should the nurse implement first?

A. Instruct the caregiver to offer a glass of warm prune juice at mealtimes.
B. Notify the HCP and request a prescription for a stool softener.
C. Assess the client's medical record to determine his normal bowel pattern.
D. Instruct the caregiver to increase the client's fluids to five 8-ounce glasses per day.

Question

A client who has chronic obstructive pulmonary disease (COPD) is resting in a semi-Fowler's position with oxygen at 2 L/min per nasal cannula. The client develops dyspnea. Which action should the nurse take first?

A. Call the HCP.
B. Obtain a bedside pulse oximeter.
C. Raise the head of the bed higher.
D. Assess the client's vital signs.

Specific Areas of Content: Lab Values

- Know the normal ranges for commonly used laboratory tests, what variations mean, and the best nursing actions.
- Hemoglobin and hematocrit (H & H)
- White blood cells (WBCs), red blood cells (RBCs), platelets
- Electrolytes: K^+, Na^+, Ca^{2+}, Mg^{2+}, Cl^-, PO_4
- Blood urea nitrogen (BUN) and creatinine
- Relationship of Ca^{2+} and PO_4
- Arterial blood gases (ABGs)
- PT (prothrombin time), international normalized ratio (INR), partial thromboplastin time (PTT) (Don't get them confused.)
- Glycosylated Hgb (A1C)

Handwritten annotations:

GFR 125mL/min

7.0 < target   norm < 5.5%

PT: 11-17   INR: 2-3 sec. —
mechanical valve 3-4 sec
PTT/APTT: 1.5-2.5   60-90
150 > risk of bleeding
antidote heparin: protamine sulfate.
warfarine ⟷ vitamin K

Question

A client who has hyperparathyroidism is scheduled to receive a prescribed dose of oral phosphate. The nurse notes that the client serum calcium is 12.5 mg/dL. What action should the nurse take?

A. Hold the phosphate and notify the HCP.
B. Review the client's serum parathyroid hormone level.
C. Give a PRN dose of intravenous (IV) calcium per protocol.
D. Administer the dose of oral phosphate.

Question

In completing a client's perioperative routine, the nurse finds that the consent form has not been signed. The client begins to ask more questions about the surgical procedure. Which action should the nurse take?

A. Witness the client's signature on the consent form.
B. Answer the client's questions about the surgery.
C. Inform the HCP that the client has questions about the surgery.
D. Reassure the client that the surgeon will answer any questions before the anesthetic is administered.

Complementary and Alternative Therapy

Complementary and alternative therapy (CAM) is influenced by culture. It includes use of herbal medications as well as other treatments such as yoga, acupressure, acupuncture, reiki, and aromatherapy.

- Know the risks and benefits.

- Know the mechanisms of action, side effects, and drug interactions.

- Know the contraindications with traditional and other herbal medications.

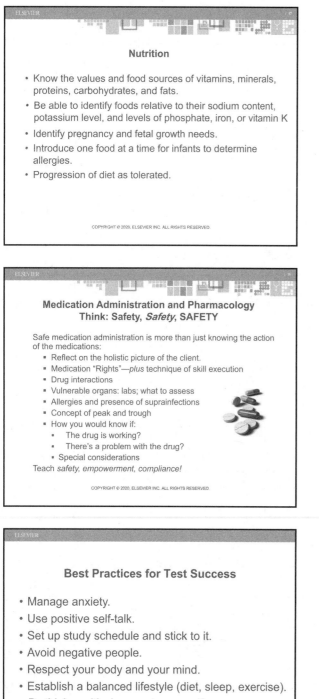

Nutrition

- Know the values and food sources of vitamins, minerals, proteins, carbohydrates, and fats.
- Be able to identify foods relative to their sodium content, potassium level, and levels of phosphate, iron, or vitamin K
- Identify pregnancy and fetal growth needs.
- Introduce one food at a time for infants to determine allergies.
- Progression of diet as tolerated.

Medication Administration and Pharmacology
Think: Safety, *Safety*, SAFETY

Safe medication administration is more than just knowing the action of the medications:
- Reflect on the holistic picture of the client.
- Medication "Rights"—*plus* technique of skill execution
- Drug interactions
- Vulnerable organs: labs; what to assess
- Allergies and presence of suprainfections
- Concept of peak and trough
- How you would know if:
  - The drug is working?
  - There's a problem with the drug?
  - Special considerations
Teach *safety, empowerment, compliance!*

Best Practices for Test Success

- Manage anxiety.
- Use positive self-talk.
- Set up study schedule and stick to it.
- Avoid negative people.
- Respect your body and your mind.
- Establish a balanced lifestyle (diet, sleep, exercise).
- *Do* think positively—say to yourself:

"I can be successful!"

Supplements: black licorice - used RA or expectorant. Monitor BP (HTN) and K⁺ (↓) Interact: heparin ∅

- St. Johns Wart: antidepressant ∅ compatible w/ meds

- Akanesia: cold / flu symptoms hepatotoxicity!

- Garlic: for BP / cholesterol / ↑immunity. ↑risk of bleeding— blood thinner.

- Ginger: GI symptoms— nausea. BG management ✱ bleeding risk

- Ginko: enhance memory function. ✱ bleeding risk

- Fevero: migraines. Interfere w/ coagulation.

- Turmeric: Anti-inflammatory

- Kava: Insomnia. ✱ hepatotoxicity

Trough level: make sure not elevated

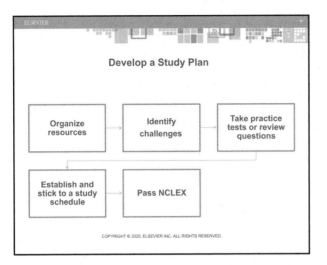

Develop a Study Plan

Organize resources → Identify challenges → Take practice tests or review questions

Establish and stick to a study schedule → Pass NCLEX

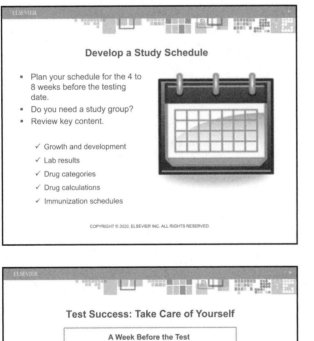

Develop a Study Schedule

- Plan your schedule for the 4 to 8 weeks before the testing date.
- Do you need a study group?
- Review key content.

  ✓ Growth and development
  ✓ Lab results
  ✓ Drug categories
  ✓ Drug calculations
  ✓ Immunization schedules

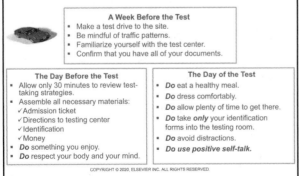

Test Success: Take Care of Yourself

A Week Before the Test
- Make a test drive to the site.
- Be mindful of traffic patterns.
- Familiarize yourself with the test center.
- Confirm that you have all of your documents.

The Day Before the Test
- Allow only 30 minutes to review test-taking strategies.
- Assemble all necessary materials:
  ✓ Admission ticket
  ✓ Directions to testing center
  ✓ Identification
  ✓ Money
- *Do* something you enjoy.
- *Do* respect your body and your mind.

The Day of the Test
- *Do* eat a healthy meal.
- *Do* dress comfortably.
- *Do* allow plenty of time to get there.
- *Do* take *only* your identification forms into the testing room.
- *Do* avoid distractions.
- *Do use positive self-talk.*

During the Exam

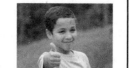

- Breathe deeply and regularly.

- Continue the positive self-talk.

- Be in the moment—**no regrets!**

- **Do not** allow the number of questions to influence your level of self-confidence.

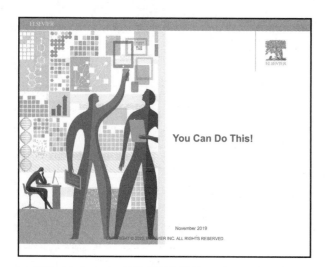

You Can Do This!

November 2019

Legal Aspects and Leadership Role of the Registered Nurse

2

Legal Systems

- Civil law is concerned with the protection of the client's private rights.
- Criminal law deals with the rights of individuals and society as defined by legislative laws.

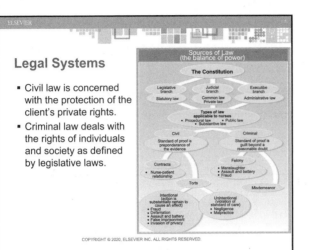

Nursing Negligence and Malpractice

Nursing Negligence	Nursing Malpractice
Failure to exercise the proper degree of care required by the circumstances that a reasonable, prudent person would exercise under the circumstances to avoid harming others (careless act)	Failure to use that degree of care that a reasonable, prudent nurse would use under the same or similar circumstance (professional negligence)

Malpractice is found when:
- The nurse owed a duty to the client.
- The nurse did not carry out that duty or breached that duty.
- The client was injured.
- The nurse's failure to carry out that duty caused the client's injury.

Standards of Care

- Nurses are required to follow standards of care, which originate in Nurse Practice Acts; state and federal law (US) and provincial, territorial, and federal laws (Canada); accreditation recommendations; the guidelines of professional organizations; and the written policy and procedures of the healthcare agency.
- Nurses are responsible for performing procedures correctly and exercising professional judgment when implementing healthcare providers' prescriptions.
- Nurses retain the accountability and responsibility for care that is delegated.

Question

The unlicensed assistive personnel (UAP) reports to the staff nurse that a client who had surgery 4 hours ago has had a decrease in blood pressure (BP), from 150/80 to 110/70, in the past hour. The nurse advises the UAP to check the client's dressing for excess drainage and report the findings to the nurse. Which factor is most important to consider when assessing the legal ramifications of this situation?

A. The parameters of the state's or province's nurse practice act
B. The need to complete an adverse occurrence report
C. Hospital protocol regarding the frequency of vital sign assessment every hour postoperatively
D. The healthcare provider's prescription for changing the postoperative dressing

Question

The newly licensed nurse overhears two nurses talking in the elevator about a client who will lose her leg because of negligence of the staff. Which action by the newly licensed nurse should be implemented first?

A. Monitor the nurses closely for further occurrences.
B. Advise them to cease their communication.
C. Inform the nurse manager of the conversation.
D. Submit an occurrence or variance report.

Practice Issues

- Nurses must follow the healthcare provider's prescription unless the nurse believes that it is in error, violates hospital policy, or is harmful to the client.
- The nurse will make a formal report explaining the refusal.
- The nurse should file an incident (occurrence; variance) report in any situation that will potentially cause harm to a client.

Advance Directives (AD)

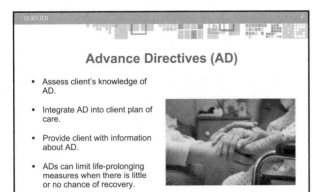

- Assess client's knowledge of AD.

- Integrate AD into client plan of care.

- Provide client with information about AD.

- ADs can limit life-prolonging measures when there is little or no chance of recovery.

- The client must receive AD information or review ADs on admission.

Advance Directives (AD)

Living Will (LW)

LW is a written document that directs treatment in accordance with a client's wishes in the event of a terminal illness or condition.

Durable Power of Attorney for Health Care

A client appoints a representative (healthcare proxy) to make healthcare decisions based on the client's wishes.

Question

An awake, alert client with impending pulmonary edema is brought to the emergency department. The client provides the nurse with a copy of a living will that states that "no invasive" medical procedures should be used to "keep her alive." The healthcare team is questioning whether the client should be intubated. Which information should guide the team's decision?

A. The living will removes the obligation to the client in any medical decision-making.

B. The client is awake and alert, which makes the living will irrelevant and nonbinding.

C. Lifesaving measures do not have to be explained to the client because of the signed living will.

D. The family should be contacted to determine who has durable power of attorney for health care for the client.

Restraints/Safety Reminder Devices (SRDs)

- Used *only* to ensure the physical safety of the client or of other residents when less restrictive interventions fail

- Must have a written prescription from a healthcare provider; must reassess prescription (i.e., at 8 or 24 hours).

- Nurse must follow agency policy and procedure to restrain any client.

Applying Physical Restraints:

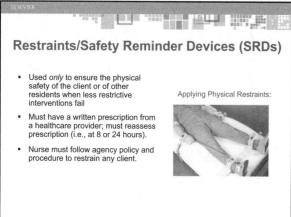

Restraints/Safety Reminder Devices (SRDs)

- Documentation of restraint use and of follow-up assessments must detail the attempts to use less restrictive interventions.

- Liability for improper or unlawful restraint lies with the nurse and healthcare facility.

- The nurse must ensure that the UAP working under the nurse's supervision uses restraints properly and according to healthcare facility procedures.

Question

A family member of a client who is in a Posey vest restraint (safety reminder device) asks why the restraint was applied. Which response should the nurse make?

A. The restraint was prescribed by the healthcare provider.

B. There is not enough staff to keep the client safe all the time.

C. The other clients are upset when the client wanders at night.

D. The client's actions place the client at high risk for self-harm.

Legal Aspects of Mental Health

- Admissions
  - Involuntary
  - Emergency
- Client rights
- Competency

Question

What nursing action has the highest priority when admitting a client to a psychiatric unit on an involuntary basis?

A. Reassure the client that this admission is only for a limited amount of time.

B. Offer the client and family the opportunity to share their feelings about the admission.

C. Determine the behaviors that resulted in the need for admission.

D. Advise the client about the legal rights of all hospitalized clients.

Confidential Health Care

- Confidentiality is the right of all clients. The American Nurses Association Code of Ethics for Nurses and the Canadian Nurses Association Code of Ethics for Registered nurses assert the duty of the nurse to protect confidentiality of clients.

- The Health Insurance Portability and Accountability Act of 1996 (HIPAA) established standards for the verbal, written, and electronic exchange of private health information.

- The Personal Information Protection and Electronic Documents Act (PIPEDA) (Canada) is federal legislation that protects personal information, including health information. PIPEDA delineates how private-sector organizations may collect, use, or disclose personal information.

BUN, creatinine, glucose differ between U.S / Canada

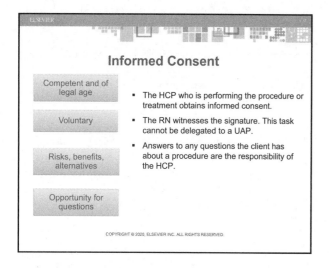

Informed Consent

Competent and of legal age

Voluntary

Risks, benefits, alternatives

Opportunity for questions

- The HCP who is performing the procedure or treatment obtains informed consent.
- The RN witnesses the signature. This task cannot be delegated to a UAP.
- Answers to any questions the client has about a procedure are the responsibility of the HCP.

Question

The nurse enters the room of a preoperative client to obtain the client's signature on the surgical consent form. Which question is most important for the nurse to ask the client?

A. "When did the surgeon explain the procedure to you?"
B. "Is any member of your family going to be here during your surgery?"
C. "Have you been instructed in postoperative activities and restrictions?"
D. "Have you received any preoperative pain medication?"

Good Samaritan Laws

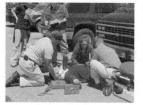

- Limit liability if a nurse offers assistance at the scene of an accident
- Provide only care that is consistent with the nurse's level of expertise
- Nurse is required to deliver care in a "reasonable and prudent manner."

Abuse

- The nurse has legal responsibilities related to reporting incidences of abuse, neglect, or violence.

- Healthcare professionals who do not report suspected abuse or neglect are liable for civil or criminal legal action.

- Obvious physical injury or neglect (e.g., evidence of malnutrition or presence of bruising on the extremities or trunk) are signs of possible abuse.

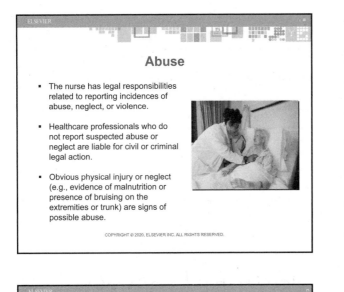

Question

Which assignment should the nurse delegate to a UAP in an acute care setting?

A. Checking blood glucose hourly for a client with a continuous insulin drip

B. Giving PO medications left at the bedside for the client to take after eating

C. Taking vital signs for an older client with left humeral and left tibial fractures

D. Replacing a client's pressure ulcer dressing that has been soiled by incontinence

Communication Skills: Types of Leadership

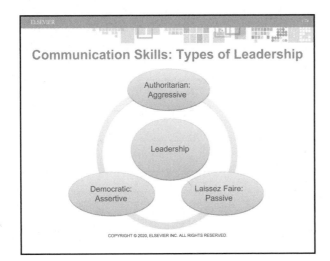

Question

The charge nurse confronts a staff nurse whose behavior has been resentful and negative since a change in unit policy was announced. The staff nurse states, "Don't blame me; nobody likes this idea." Which is the charge nurse's priority action?

A. Confront the other staff members involved in the change of unit policy.
B. Call a unit meeting to review the reasons the change was made.
C. Develop a written unit policy for the expression of complaints.
D. Encourage the nurse to be accountable for her own behavior.

Delegation and Supervision Skills

The process by which responsibility and authority—but **not accountability**—are transferred to another individual.

The nursing process or any activity requiring nursing judgment may not be delegated to the unlicensed assistive personnel (UAP).

Five Rights of Delegation
1. Right task
2. Right circumstance
3. Right person
4. Right direction/communication
5. Right supervision

Supervision
- Direction/guidance
- Evaluation/monitoring
- Follow-up

Handwritten notes:
Task: routine / non-invasive
Circumstance: resource availability
Stable pt
Person: scope + competence

Supervision: Monitoring

Delegation Skills

RN Responsibilities
- Determine client needs and when to delegate.
- Ensure availability of delegatee.
- Evaluate outcomes of and maintain accountability for delegated responsibility.

Delegatee Responsibility
- Accept activities based on own competence level.
- Maintain competence for delegated responsibility.
- Maintain accountability for delegated activity.

Question

The charge nurse is making assignments for each of four staff members, including a registered nurse (RN), a licensed practical nurse (PN), and two unlicensed assistive personnel (UAPs). Which task is best to assign to the PN?

A. Maintain a 24-hour urine collection.
B. Wean a client from a mechanical ventilator.
C. Perform sterile wound irrigation.
D. Obtain scheduled vital signs.

Question

Which situation warrants a variance (incident) report by the nurse?

A. A client refuses to take prescribed medication.
B. A client's status improves before completion of the course of medication.
C. A client has an allergic reaction to a prescribed medication.
D. A client received medication prescribed for another client.

Effective Team Communication

Communication focuses on:
- Team building
- Facilitating collaboration
- Consulting
- Delegating
- Supervising
- Leading and managing

Effective Team Communication

- Lateral violence refers to acts that occur among colleagues, whereas bullying is described as acts perpetrated by one in a higher level of authority that occur over time (ANA, 2015).
- These may affect client safety.
- Examples of the impact on client safety could include:
  - Delayed medication administration caused by failure to notify the nurse responsible for giving the medication of a change
  - Delayed notification of a change in prescriptions by the HCP
  - Nurse omits pertinent information re: client's care or prescriptions

---

Effective Team Communication

- Best practices include:
  - Communicate clearly.
  - Treat others with respect.
  - Avoid gossip.
  - Rely on facts.
  - Collaborate.
  - Offer assistance when needed.
  - Speak directly to the individual with whom one has an issue.

Handoff Communication

- Important client information is shared at pertinent points of care.

- Ensures continuity of care and client safety

- Improves communication and appropriate delegation

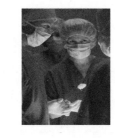

Question

The nurse is preparing for change of shift. Which action by the nurse is characteristic of ineffective handoff communication?

A. The nurse states to the nurse coming on duty: "The client is anxious about pain after surgery. Review the information I provided about how to use an incentive spirometer."

B. The nurse refers to the electronic medical record (EMR) to review the client's medication administration record.

C. During rounds, the nurse talks about the problem the UAP created by not performing a fingerstick blood glucose test on the client.

D. Before giving report, the nurse performs rounds on assigned clients so that there is less likelihood of interruption during handoff.

S-BAR

S-BAR is an interdisciplinary communication strategy that promotes effective communication between caregivers.

I: Introduction

S = **SITUATION:** State the issue or problem.

B = **BACKGROUND:** Provide the client's history.

A = **ASSESSMENT:** Give the most recent vital signs and current findings.

R = **RECOMMENDATIONS:** State what should be done.

R: Repeat

Culturally Sensitive Care

- The client's culture, religious group, and country of origin influence his or her healthcare beliefs.
- The cultural assessment answers questions such as:
  - Primary language spoken
  - Pain management expectations
  - Support systems
  - Feelings regarding gender of caregiver
  - Whether client gives family members control over healthcare decisions
- Explain to client and interpreter that confidentiality will be maintained.
- Value different styles of communication used by clients, families, and healthcare providers.
- Employ culturally relevant and language appropriate teaching materials and techniques.

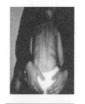

Question

The charge nurse is planning client assignments for the shift. The care team includes a registered nurse (RN), a licensed practical nurse (PN), and unlicensed assistive personnel (UAP) on the care team. Which client(s) are appropriate to be assigned to the PN? (Select all that apply.)

A. A client scheduled for a STAT CAT x-ray after a fall from a stretcher

B. A client receiving IV vancomycin through a peripherally inserted catheter (PICC) line

C. A client with sickle cell crisis who was transferred from the ICU to the acute care area and who is receiving hydromorphone via a patient-controlled analgesia (PCA) pump

D. A client with a pressure ulcer who was prescribed negative pressure (wound VAC) care

E. A postoperative client who has been prescribed 2 units of packed red blood cells

Question

A charge nurse is making assignments for five clients. The nursing team has an RN, a PN, and two UAPs. Which client(s) are appropriate to assign to the RN? (Select all that apply.)

A. A client from the previous shift with unstable angina

B. A client with a stage 3 pressure ulcer who needs a bed bath

C. A client with an enteral feeding absorbing at 30 mL/h

D. A cardiotomy client who is day 2 postoperative and who has chest tubes

E. A client with quadriplegia for whom urinary catherization is prescribed

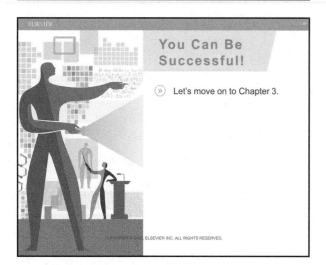

You Can Be Successful!

» Let's move on to Chapter 3.

Clinical Concepts and Mechanisms of Disease

3

Operative Care: Preoperative Care

Preparation

- Obtain a complete history, including the following:
  - Physical assessment
  - List of current medications (prescriptions, OTC, complementary) and allergies
  - Previous surgical experiences (response to anesthetic)
  - Signed consent (confirm informed consent **before** client is sedated)
  - Confirm labs and diagnostics
  - Skin preparation
  - Preop checklist and preprocedure verification

Preoperative Care

Preoperative Teaching

- Diet restrictions (typically NPO [nothing by mouth] after midnight before surgery)

- Teach coughing and deep breathing, incentive spirometry.

- Review methods of pain control.

- Complete preoperative verification process.

Postoperative Care

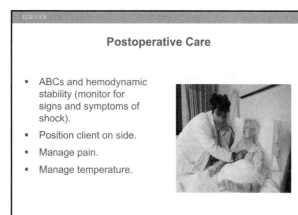

- ABCs and hemodynamic stability (monitor for signs and symptoms of shock).
- Position client on side.
- Manage pain.
- Manage temperature.

Nursing and Collaborative Care

- Urinary retention
  - Check for distention.
  - UTI
  - Remove urinary catheter POD #1/POD#2.
- Pulmonary problems
  - Check breath sounds.
  - Check O_2 saturation.
- Bowel sounds
  - Decreased peristalsis
  - Paralytic ileus
- Wound management
  - Incisions, drains, skin integrity
  - Wound dehiscence or evisceration
- Venous thromboembolism (VTE)

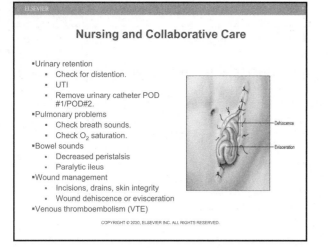

Dehiscence

Evisceration

Assumed paramater orders for opioids.

Question

A 72-year-old client returned from surgery 6 hours ago. The client received hydromorphone 2 mg IV 30 minutes ago for pain rating 8/10. The family member requests her father be checked immediately. On arrival to the room, the nurse finds the client difficult to arouse, with a respiration rate of 6. Which is the priority nursing action?

A. Elevate the head of the bed.

B. Administer naloxone 0.4 mg IV.

C. Assess breath sounds.

D. Check vital signs and pulse oximetry.

Pain

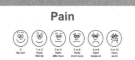

- Pain management is client centered.
- Pain is whatever the client says it is, existing whenever he or she says it does.
- Nurses have both a legal and ethical responsibility for managing clients' pain and suffering (be aware of any personal bias or misconceptions about pain management).

Pain Assessment and Management

Assessment includes:
- **P**: precipitating or palliative
- **Q**: quality
- **R**: relief measures/region (location)
- **S**: severity (using a scale appropriate for age and client condition: numerical, descriptive, a set of faces with expressions)
- **T**: timing (onset, duration)
- **U**: effect of pain on client's ability to perform ADLs
- Observe for nonverbal behaviors, which may indicate pain (moaning, grimacing, clenched teeth, pacing, or inactivity).
- Wong-Baker FACES Pain Rating Scale recommended for persons 3 years of age and older.
- Assess personal cultural, spiritual, and ethical beliefs that may influence the perception of pain.

Pain Assessment and Management

- Consider special populations: palliative care, end of life.
- Documentation includes pain assessment data (pre- and post-intervention rating), interventions (both nonpharmacological and pharmacological), and client teaching.
- Controlled substance disposal must be documented per regulatory guidelines (ask another nurse to witness the waste of a pill fragment, discarded injection contents, or discarded liquid contents).

Nonpharmacological Noninvasive Pain Relief Techniques

- Repositioning
- Cutaneous stimulation: heat and cold application, massage therapy, transcutaneous electrical nerve stimulation (TENS)
- Relaxation techniques
- Guided imagery
- Complementary and alternative medicine (CAM) (e.g., acupressure or yoga)

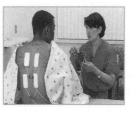

Oucher (Age 3-12) pain scale
- Cultural photo scale

Nonverbals: men, children, cultures.

Ø use cold: Sickle cell, Raynauds

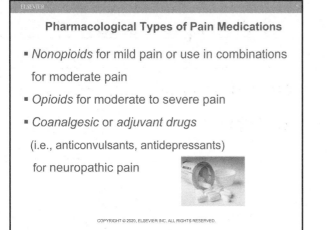

Pharmacological Types of Pain Medications

- *Nonopioids* for mild pain or use in combinations for moderate pain
- *Opioids* for moderate to severe pain
- *Coanalgesic* or *adjuvant drugs* (i.e., anticonvulsants, antidepressants) for neuropathic pain

---

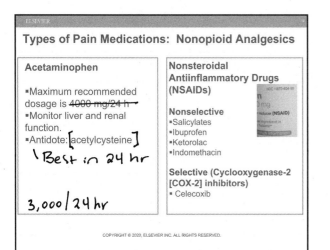

Types of Pain Medications: Nonopioid Analgesics

Acetaminophen	Nonsteroidal Antiinflammatory Drugs (NSAIDs)
▪Maximum recommended dosage is 4000 mg/24 h	**Nonselective**
▪Monitor liver and renal function.	▪Salicylates
▪Antidote: [acetylcysteine]	▪Ibuprofen
	▪Ketorolac
	▪Indomethacin
	Selective (Cyclooxygenase-2 [COX-2] inhibitors)
	▪ Celecoxib

Types of Pain Medications: Opioid Analgesics and Adjuvant Drugs

Mu Agonists
- Morphine
- Hydromorphone
- Meperidine
- Methadone
- Levorphanol
- Fentanyl
- Oxycodone
- Hydrocodone
- Codeine

Partial Agonists
- Buprenorphine hydrochloride
- Butorphanol
- Nalbuphine hydrochloride
- Pentazocine hydrochloride

Adjuvant Drugs (used for neuropathic pain)
- Anticonvulsants, antidepressants, anesthetics
  - Prescribed alone or in combination with opioids
- Corticosteroids

Handwritten notes:

Ibuprofen ↓ effectiveness of ACE inhibitors.

acetaminophen toxicity: Ø early symptoms. Blood draw needed.

· Nonselectives do NOT protect prostaglandins — erodes

· Salicylates: Aspirin — avoid
    - <12 age. May Kawasaki, Rheumatic fever, Idiopathic Arthritis

Notes near Acetaminophen box:
↳ Best in 24 hr
3,000/24 hr

Nonpharmacological Invasive Pain Relief Techniques

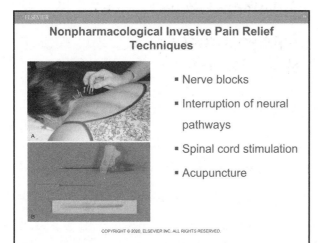

- Nerve blocks
- Interruption of neural pathways
- Spinal cord stimulation
- Acupuncture

Question

A client has an order for hydromorphone intravenous (IV) push 1 mg every 3 hours. The drug is available as 4 mg/mL. The nurse administers _____ mL of hydromorphone for one dose. (Fill in the blank.)

0.25 mL

Fluids and Electrolytes

Fluid Balance

- Changes in osmolarity cause shifts in fluid. The osmolarity of the extracellular fluid (ECF) is almost entirely due to sodium.
- The osmolarity of intracellular fluid (ICF) is related to many particles, with potassium being the primary electrolyte.
- The pressures in the ECF and the ICF are almost identical. If either ECF or ICF changes in concentration, fluid shifts from the area of lesser concentration to the area of greater concentration.

Fluids and Electrolytes

Fluid Volume Excess

Causes
CHF (most common), renal failure, cirrhosis, overhydration

Symptoms
Peripheral edema, periorbital edema, elevated BP, dyspnea, altered LOC

Lab findings
↓ BUN, ↓ Hgb, ↓ Hct, ↓ serum osmolality, ↓ urine specific gravity

Treatment
Diuretics, fluid restrictions, weigh daily, monitor K+

Fluid Volume Deficit

Causes
Inadequate fluid intake, hemorrhage, vomiting, diarrhea, massive edema

Symptoms
Weight loss, oliguria, postural hypotension

Lab findings
↑ BUN and ↑ or normal creatinine, ↑ Hgb, ↑ Hct, ↑ urine specific gravity

Treatment
Strict intake and output (I&O), replace with isotonic fluids, monitor BP, weigh daily

Types of IV Fluids

- *Isotonic* fluids expand the extracellular fluid volume (osmolarity between 250 and 300 mOsm/L): 0.9% normal saline (NS), LR (lactated Ringer's solution).

- *Hypotonic* fluids move water into the cell by osmosis, causing them to swell (osmolarity less than 250 mOsm/L): 0.45NS.

- *Hypertonic* fluids pull fluid from cells, causing them to shrink (osmolarity >300 mOsm/L): D10; 3% Saline, D5 in 0.45NS.

Sodium

Sodium: responsible for skeletal muscle contraction, cardiac contraction, nerve impulse transmission, and normal osmolarity and volume of the ECF

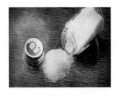

Aldosterone antagonist:
Spironolactone.
Na⁺ 132: Fluid restriction

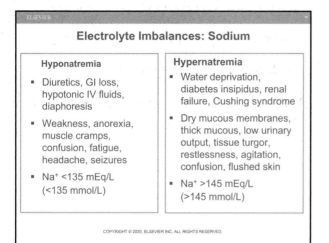

Electrolyte Imbalances: Sodium

Hyponatremia

- Diuretics, GI loss, hypotonic IV fluids, diaphoresis
- Weakness, anorexia, muscle cramps, confusion, fatigue, headache, seizures
- Na^+ <135 mEq/L (<135 mmol/L)

Hypernatremia

- Water deprivation, diabetes insipidus, renal failure, Cushing syndrome
- Dry mucous membranes, thick mucous, low urinary output, tissue turgor, restlessness, agitation, confusion, flushed skin
- Na^+ >145 mEq/L (>145 mmol/L)

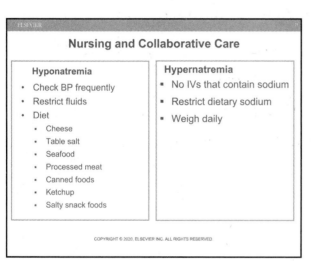

Nursing and Collaborative Care

Hyponatremia

- Check BP frequently
- Restrict fluids
- Diet
  - Cheese
  - Table salt
  - Seafood
  - Processed meat
  - Canned foods
  - Ketchup
  - Salty snack foods

Hypernatremia

- No IVs that contain sodium
- Restrict dietary sodium
- Weigh daily

Handwritten notes:

Conibaptan ⎱
            ⎰ Sodium replenishers
Tolvatan ⎱ Na^+ goes up

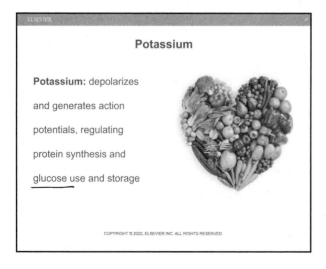

Potassium

Potassium: depolarizes and generates action potentials, regulating protein synthesis and glucose use and storage

Electrolyte Imbalances: Potassium

Hypokalemia

- Diuretics, vomiting, diarrhea, Cushing syndrome, gastric suction
- K+ <3.5 mmol/L (mEq/L)
- Rapid, thready pulse, flat T waves, fatigue, anorexia, muscle cramps

Hyperkalemia

- Oliguria, acidosis, renal failure, Addison disease
- K+ >5 mmol/L (mEq/L)
- Tall tented T waves, bradycardia, muscle weakness

Nursing and Collaborative Management

Hypokalemia

- IV potassium
- Diet: foods high in K+
  - Oranges
  - Bananas
  - Apricots
  - Cantaloupe
  - Legumes
  - Leafy vegetables
  - Potatoes
  - Meat

Hyperkalemia

- 10% to 20% glucose with regular insulin
- Sodium polystyrene sulfonate is used to treat hyperkalemia
- IV loop diuretics
- Renal dialysis

Calcium

Calcium: maintains bone strength and density, activates enzymes, allows skeletal and cardiac muscle contraction, controls nerve impulse transmission, and allows for blood clotting

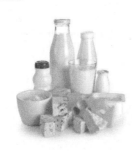

Handwritten notes:

mild — moderate — severe
5-6   7-10   10 >

Sodium polystyrene sulfonate
Patiromer : for CKD Ø impact Na⁺
"K⁺ excelate"

Beta - Blockers ⎫ Potential to
ARBS   ⎬ Raise K⁺
Digoxin   ⎬
Heparin   ⎬
ACE Inhibitors   ⎭

CKD → ∅ Vitamin D → ↓Ca⁺

hypocalcemia: can lead to laryngeal
Spasm. "Stridor": harsh vibratory

Electrolyte Imbalances: Calcium

Hypocalcemia

- Renal failure, hypoparathyroidism malabsorption, pancreatitis, alkalosis
- Ca++ <2.25 mmol/L (<9 mEq/L)
- + Chvostek sign, +Trousseau sign, diarrhea, numbness, and convulsions

Hypercalcemia

- Hyperparathyroidism, malignant bone disease, excessive supplementation
- Ca^{2+} >2.75 mmol/L (>10.5 mEq/L)
- Muscle weakness, constipation, nausea and vomiting, dysrhythmias, behavioral changes

Nursing and Collaborative Management

Hypocalcemia

- Administer calcium supplements.
- Give IV calcium slowly.
- Encourage calcium-rich foods, vitamin D, protein.
- For acute hypocalcemia, keep a tracheostomy tray and resuscitation bag at bedside in case of laryngeal spasms.

Hypercalcemia

- Limit vitamin D intake.
- Avoid calcium-based antacids.
- Administer calcitonin to reduce calcium.
- Renal dialysis may be required.

Magnesium

Magnesium: controls skeletal muscle contraction, carbohydrate metabolism, adenosine triphosphate [ATP] formation, vitamin activation, and cell growth

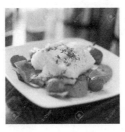

Electrolyte Imbalances: Magnesium

Hypomagnesemia	Hypermagnesemia
▪Alcoholism, malabsorption, diabetic ketoacidosis, diuretics	▪Renal failure, adrenal insufficiency, excess replacement
▪Mg^{2+} <0.65 mmol/L (<1.3 mEq/L)	▪Mg^{2+} >1.05 mmol/L (>2.1 mEq/L)
▪Skeletal muscle weakness	▪Bradycardia
▪Hyperactive deep tendon reflexes	▪Peripheral vasodilation
▪Numbness and tingling	▪Hypotension
▪Painful muscle contractions	▪Prolonged PR interval with a widened QRS complex
▪Decreased gastrointestinal (GI) motility, nausea	▪Decreased to absent deep tendon reflexes

Nursing and Collaborative Management

Hypomagnesemia

- Give oral supplements.
- Increase dietary intake of magnesium.
- IV magnesium
- Via infusion pump
- Monitor vital signs.

Hypermagnesemia

- No magnesium drugs for CKD clients
- IV administration of calcium chloride or calcium gluconate

Phosphorous

Phosphorous: activates vitamins and enzymes, forms ATP for energy supplies, assists in cell growth and metabolism, maintains acid-base balance and calcium homeostasis

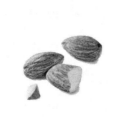

Norm: 1.3 - 2.1

Mag sulfate to prevent seizures 4-8 level in preeclampsia

① Sign mag toxicity: loss of DTR.

Torsades de pointes: hypomag.

Electrolyte Imbalances: Phosphorous

Hypophosphatemia

- Alcohol withdrawal, diabetic ketoacidosis, respiratory alkalosis
- Phosphate <0.97 mmol/L (<3.0 mg/dL)
- ↓ Cardiac output, weak peripheral pulses
- Skeletal muscle weakness

Hyperphosphatemia

- Renal failure, excess intake
- Phosphate >1.45 mmol/L (>4.5 mg/dL)
- Symptoms include signs of hypocalcemia.

Nursing and Collaborative Management

Hypophosphatemia

- Oral supplementation
- Diet high in phosphorus

Hyperphosphatemia

- Phosphate binders
- Diet low in phosphorus

Question

A client is receiving an infusion of dobutamine hydrochloride. The order reads: Infuse dobutamine IV at 5 mcg/kg/min. 500 mg in 250 mL D$_5$W. The client weighs 65 kg. Calculate the flow rate in mL/hour.

_____9.75_____ mL/hour

Handwritten notes:

5mcg (65kg) 1 min

$$\frac{325 mcg}{min} \times \frac{1 mg}{1000 mcg} \times \frac{250 mL}{500 mg} \times \frac{60 min}{1 hr}$$

4,875,000

500,000   9.75

Question

Which laboratory result for a preoperative client should prompt the nurse to contact the healthcare provider?

A. Platelet count: 151×10^9/L (151,000/mm³)
B. White blood cell (WBC) count: 85×10^9/L (8500/mm³)
C. Serum potassium level: 2.8 mEq/L (mmol/L)
D. Urine specific gravity: 1.031

Acid Base

Acid-Base Balance

pH
- Normal = 7.35 to 7.45
- <7.35 = acidosis
- >7.45 = alkalosis

pCO_2
- Normal = 35 to 45 mm Hg
- >45 = acidosis
- <35 = alkalosis

HCO_3
- Normal = 21 to 28 mEq/L
- <21 = acidosis
- >28 = alkalosis

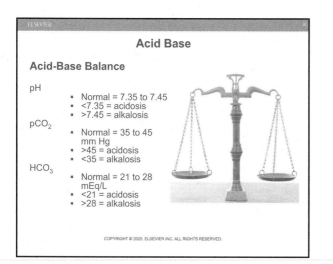

Arterial Blood Gas Interpretation Practice

pH = 7.32
pCO_2 = 50
HCO_3 = 25

This client has ___Respiratory Acidosis___ .

ELSEVIER

Arterial Blood Gas Interpretation Practice

pH = 7.28
pCO_2 = 35
HCO_3 = 18

This client has Metabolic Acidosis.

ELSEVIER

Arterial Blood Gas Interpretation Practice

pH = 7.43
pCO_2 = 40
HCO_3 = 24

This client has Normal.

ELSEVIER

Arterial Blood Gas Interpretation Practice

pH = 7.56
pCO_2 = 44
HCO_3 = 38

This client has Metabolic Alkalosis.

Arterial Blood Gas Interpretation Practice

pH = 7.33

pCO_2 = 50

HCO_3 = 29

This client has _Respiratory._ _Acidosic_

Metabolic compensation — partially.

Safety: Sentinel Events

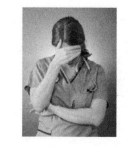

- ❖ An unexpected outcome involving a death or serious injury
- ❖ Signals the need for immediate investigation and response
- ❖ Accredited hospitals are expected to identify and respond to all sentinel events

Examples of Sentinel Events

- Client suicide
- Operative/postoperative complication
- Wrong-site surgery
- Medication error
- Client fall
- Client death or injury in restraints
- Transfusion error

Safety: Response to Sentinel Events

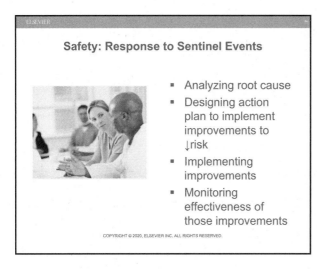

- Analyzing root cause
- Designing action plan to implement improvements to ↓risk
- Implementing improvements
- Monitoring effectiveness of those improvements

Falls: Risk Factors

Adults	Infants and Children
• Stroke	• Length of stay
• Depression	• IV or saline lock
• Mobility	• Use of antiseizure
• History of seizures, falls	medications
• Use of assistive devices	• Acute or chronic orthopedic diagnosis
• Polypharmacy	• Receiving physical or occupational therapy
• Environmental issues	• History of falls
• Forgetting or ignoring mobility issues	

Nursing and Collaborative Management

- Fall prevention
- Safety surveillance
- Assess need for pain relief, toileting, and positioning
- Frequent reorientation
- Client and family education
- Address environmental concerns
- Client sitter

High-Alert Medications

Most likely to cause significant harm to a client even when used as intended.

Types of Drugs
- Anticoagulants, narcotics and opiates, insulin, chemotherapeutic drugs, and sedatives

Types of Harm
- Hypotension, bleeding, hypoglycemia, delirium, lethargy, bradycardia

Prevention Strategies
- Built-in redundancies
- Double-checking
- Smart pumps
- Standardized or protocol-driven order sets

Death and Grief

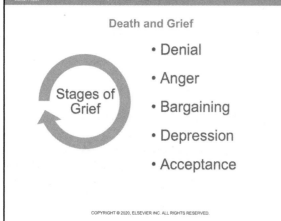

Stages of Grief

- Denial
- Anger
- Bargaining
- Depression
- Acceptance

Death and Grief

- Encourage client to express anger.
- Do not take away the defense mechanisms for coping that the client uses in crisis.
- Customs surrounding death and dying vary among cultures.
- Make every attempt to understand and accommodate the family's cultural traditions when caring for the dying client.

Infection

Infection is the invasion of the body by a pathogen.

Response to the invasion can be:

- Localized
- Systemic

Nosocomial, or hospital-acquired, infections

- Acquired as a result of exposure to a microorganism in a hospital setting

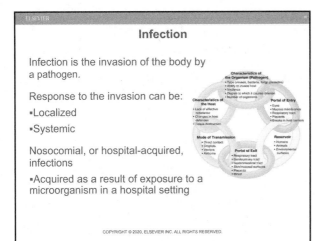

Human Immunodeficiency Virus (HIV)

Routes of Transmission

- Unprotected sexual contact
  - Most common mode of transmission
- Exposure to blood through drug-using equipment
- Perinatal transmission
  - During pregnancy
  - At the time of delivery
  - Breastfeeding

Nursing Assessment

Laboratory Testing for HIV

- Positive result on enzyme-linked immunosorbent assay (ELISA)
- Confirmed Western blot test
- Positive p24 antigen assay
- Polymerase chain reaction (PCR) (used with neonate)
- OraQuick In-Home HIV Test: Positive result is only preliminary; it must be confirmed by an HCP

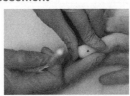

Diagnosis of AIDS

- HIV positive and a CD4+ T-cell count <200 cells/mm^3 ~~or~~ ~~an~~ opportunistic infection

AND

[handwritten note:] Category C: more resources available

Nursing Assessment

- Primary HIV infection
  - Earliest stage: begins with flulike symptoms and antibodies may develop in weeks 1 to 12
- Early (symptomatic) HIV disease signs and symptoms may not present until 10 to 14 years after initial exposure without treatment
  - Fatigue, severe weight loss, swollen glands, unexplained fever, night sweats, dry cough
- Parasites, fungi, bacteria, and viruses cause of opportunistic diseases
  - Candidiasis: lungs, bronchi, esophagus
  - Invasive cervical cancer
  - CMV
  - HIV-related encephalopathy

Nursing and Collaborative Management

- Monitor disease progression and immune function.
- Prevent development of opportunistic diseases.
- Detect and treat opportunistic diseases.
- Manage symptoms.
- Prevent or decrease complications of treatment.
- Prevent transmission of HIV.
- Encourage proper nutrition.
- Refer to mental health counseling.
- Encourage safe sex practices.

high calorie/high protein diet

HIV Drug Therapy

Initiate and monitor highly active antiretroviral therapy (HAART).

3 Goals of Drug Therapy:

- Decrease the viral load.
- Maintain or raise CD4+ T-cell counts.
- Delay the development of HIV-related symptoms and opportunistic diseases.

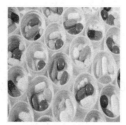

Nursing and Collaborative Management

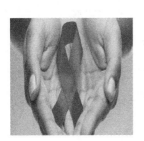

- The client should have regular blood counts to track CD4 levels and the viral load.
- Side effects are common, and there are many drug-drug interactions.

HIV Medications

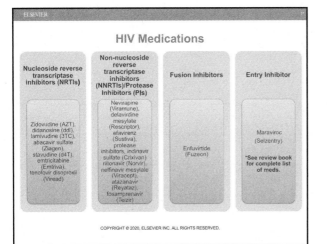

Nucleoside reverse transcriptase inhibitors (NRTIs)	Non-nucleoside reverse transcriptase inhibitors (NNRTIs)/Protease Inhibitors (PIs)	Fusion Inhibitors	Entry Inhibitor
Zidovudine (AZT), didanosine (ddI), lamivudine (3TC), abacavir sulfate (Ziagen), stavudine (d4T), emtricitabine (Emtriva), tenofovir disoproxil (Viread)	Nevirapine (Viramune), delavirdine mesylate (Rescriptor), efavirenz (Sustiva), protease inhibitors, indinavir sulfate (Crixivan) ritonavir (Norvir), nelfinavir mesylate (Viracept), atazanavir (Reyataz), fosamprenavir (Telzir)	Enfuvirtide (Fuzeon)	Maraviroc (Selzentry) *See review book for complete list of meds.

Pediatric HIV: Clinical Manifestations

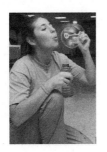

- Recurrent infections such as thrush
- Unexplained fever
- Lymphadenopathy
- Hepatosplenomegaly
- Oral candidiasis
- Failure to thrive
- Developmental delay

Treated NRTRI during pregnancy.

Nursing and Collaborative Management

- Teach transmission and control of infectious diseases.
- Safety issues include appropriate storage of special medications and equipment.
- Prevention is a key component of HIV education.
- Aggressive pain management is essential.
- Common psychosocial concerns include disclosure of the diagnosis.
- Do not administer live viruses.
- Address psychosocial concerns.
- If an HIV-infected mother is treated with zidovudine during pregnancy and the neonate is treated after birth, the probability of HIV infection of the child decreases.

Symptoms guide admin of live vaccines.

Question

A client, who is HIV positive, asks why it is necessary to have a viral load study performed every 3 to 4 months. Which information should the nurse provide?

A. To determine the progression of the disease
B. To evaluate the enzyme-linked immunosorbent assay (ELISA)
C. To monitor the effectiveness of the treatment
D. To track the effectiveness of the vaccine

① Early detection
② Safe care

Cancer

- The leading sites of primary cancer in men are the prostate, lungs, colon, and rectum. The leading sites of primary cancer in women are the breasts, lungs, colon, and rectum.
- Lung cancer is the leading cause of cancer-related deaths in both men and women.
- The incidence of cancer is higher among African Americans than among white people.

Primary Prevention
- Education about lifestyle changes and risk factors
  - Smoking/smokeless tobacco
  - Dietary habits
  - Ultraviolet radiation
  - Excessive alcohol use
- Cancer risk assessment
- Genetic counseling

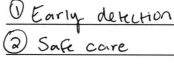

Cancer

Health Promotion

•The National Cancer Institute has recommended including at least five servings of fruits and vegetables in the daily diet. In addition are the following recommendations:

- Eat foods from protein sources such as lean meat, fish, and skinned poultry.
- Choose low-fat dairy products, including white cheese rather than yellow.
- Eat whole grains.
- Include beans in the diet.
- Limit intake of saturated fat and added sugars.

Contact the HCP if the client has:

•Changes in bowel or bladder habits
•A sore that does not heal
•Unusual bleeding or discharge
•Thickening or lump in breast or elsewhere, etc.
•Indigestion or difficulty swallowing
•Obvious change in warts or moles
•Nagging cough or hoarseness

Cancer

Screening Recommendations

•Breast
•Cervix
•Colorectal
•Endometrial
•Lung
•Prostate
•Testicular

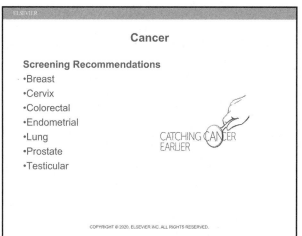

CATCHING CANCER EARLIER

Cancer

Diagnosis of Cancer

•Considerations for use in the diagnosis of cancer

- Biopsy
- Endoscope
- Diagnostic imaging
- Radioisotope studies
- Laboratory tests
  - Alkaline phosphatase blood levels
  - Calcitonin
  - Carcinoembryonic antigen (CEA)
  - Tumor markers
  - Stool for occult blood

Colorectal screening: age 45

PSA: prostate cancer

Cancer Therapies

- **Surgery:** may be preventative, diagnostic, curative, or palliative
  - Nursing considerations: teaching specific to surgery
- ✱ **External Radiation** ✱
  - Keep skin dry
  - Do not apply lotions, ointments, creams, and powders in marked areas. Any lotions used must be prescribed by the physician.
  - Protect the radiated area from direct sunlight.
  - Instruct the client not to remove the markings.
  - Avoid applications of heat or cold.
  - Encourage 2 to 3 liters of fluids per day.
  - Encourage a diet high in protein and calories.

Cancer Therapies

- ✱ **Internal Radiation** ✱
  - Sealed radioactive materials (radioactive implant [brachytherapy])
    - Client in private room
    - Limit time with client.
    - Wear radioactive badge.
    - Keep lead-lined container in room.
    - Wear dosimeter film badge when providing care.
  - Unsealed internal radiation: e.g., radioactive iodine for thyroid cancer
    - Client in a private room
    - Limit time spent with client.
    - Wear dosimeter when in client room.

Question

The charge nurse is assigning rooms for four new clients. Only one private room is available in the oncology unit. Which client should be placed in the private room?

A. The client with ovarian cancer who is receiving chemotherapy

B. The client with breast cancer who is receiving external beam radiation

C. The client with prostate cancer who has just had a transurethral resection

D. The client with cervical cancer who is receiving intracavity radiation

Handwritten notes:

① Care post-chemo
② Management
high protein / high calorie
★ Fatigue

Common w/ cervical cancer

Chemotherapy

Strict guidelines must be followed!

These drugs normally are administered by chemotherapy-certified nurses.

Pregnant nurses should not administer most of these agents.

Wear personal protective equipment for hazardous drug handling.

➤Gowns: disposable, made of fabric that has low permeability to the agents in use, with closed front and cuffs

➤Gloves: powder free, labeled for use with chemotherapy drugs, latex, nitrile, or neoprene

---

Chemotherapeutic Agents

Monitor for extravasation during infusion, and notify the HCP immediately if this occurs.

Types of IV access devices used for administration:
- Hickman
- Broviac
- Port-a-cath

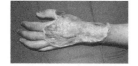
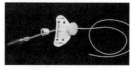

vesicants

Chemotherapeutic Agents

Side effects to monitor after chemotherapy
- Leukopenia (WBC <4000 mm)
- Neutropenia
- Anemia
- Thrombocytopenia
- Stomatitis
- Alopecia
- Anorexia
- Diarrhea
- Tumor lysis syndrome

Question

The complete blood count (CBC) results for a client receiving chemotherapy are hemoglobin 85 mmol/L (8.5 g/dL); hematocrit, 32%; WBC count, 6.5 × 109/L (6500 cells/mm^3). Which meal choice is best for this client?

A. Grilled chicken, rice, fresh fruit salad, milk
B. Broiled steak, whole wheat rolls, spinach salad, coffee
C. Smoked ham, mashed potatoes, applesauce, iced tea
D. Tuna noodle casserole, garden salad, lemonade

Question

The nurse is caring for a client who is 24 hours postprocedure for a hemicolectomy with a temporary colostomy placement. The nurses assesses the client's stoma, which is dry and dark blue. Which action should the nurse take based on this finding?

A. Notify the healthcare provider of the finding.
B. Document the finding in the client record.
C. Replace the pouch system over the stoma.
D. Place petrolatum gauze dressing on the stoma.

Question

After the change-of-shift report, the nurse reviews assignments. Which client should the nurse assess first?

A. The elderly client receiving palliative care for heart failure who complains of constipation and nervousness
B. The adult client who is 48 hours postoperative for a colectomy and who is reported to be having nausea and vomiting
C. The middle-aged client with chronic renal failure whose urinary catheter has been draining 95 mL for 8 hours
D. The client who is 2 days postoperative for a thoracotomy and who has chest tubes, is on oxygen at 3 L/min, and has a respiratory rate of 12 breaths/min

Question

A practical nurse (PN) is assigned to care for an 82-year-old client who had a total right hip replacement with cement 2 days ago. Which observation(s) should the PN immediately report to the RN? (Select all that apply.)

A. The client complains of incisional pain, rating it an 8 on a scale of 0 to 10.

B. The client has had a change in orientation to person but not to time or place.

C. Swelling and redness have developed in the client's lower left leg.

D. The LPN emptied 15 mL of bloody drainage from the Jackson-Pratt drain.

E. The client's last set of vital signs was temperature 37.9°C (100.2°F), pulse 87, respirations 12, blood pressure 108/74, and O_2 saturation 93%.

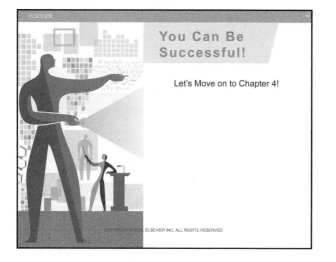

You Can Be Successful!

Let's Move on to Chapter 4!

4 Advanced Clinical Concepts and Disaster Management

ELSEVIER

Acute Conditions: Shock

Stages of Shock

Stage 1: Nonprogressive

★ Restlessness

MAP ↓ 10 to 15 mm Hg from baseline

↑ Heart rate

↓ Urine output (oliguria)

Pulse oximetry 90% to 95%

↑ Respiratory rate

Neurogenic shock: HR goes ↓

ELSEVIER

Acute Conditions: Shock

Stages of Shock

Stage 2: Progressive

Pallor/cyanosis of mucosa/nail beds

MAP ↓ >20 mm Hg

↓ pH, ↑ lactate

Rapid, weak thread pulse

Cool, moist skin

Pulse oximetry 75% to 80%

Anuria

Stage 3: Refractory

Rapid LOC change

Toxic metabolite release leads to unresponsiveness to shock correction

Slow, shallow respirations

Pulse oximetry <70%

Multiple organ dysfunction syndrome (MODS) 2 ≥ Fail

ELSEVIER

Types of Shock

Hypovolemic	Vasogenic (Anaphylactic, Neurogenic, Septic)	Cardiogenic	Obstructive
• ↓ Circulating volume related to internal or external blood loss or dehydration • Older adults at risk related to diuretic therapy, ↓ thirst reflex, anticoagulation therapy	• Excessive vasodilation and impaired distribution of blood flow • Older adult risk related to ↓ immune response, malignancies, malnutrition	• Pump failure • Results in ↓ cardiac output and MAP • Older adult risk related to diabetes mellitus, cardiomyopathies, cognitive impairment • MI is the most common cause	• Physical obstruction that impedes filling and pumping of the heart • Pericarditis, cardiac tamponade • Older adult risk related to autoimmune disorders, malignancies, pulmonary hypertension

Anaphylaxis: (1) epi, (2) steroids, (3) Benadryl.

Cardiogenic: (+) inotrope ↑ contractility. (−) ↓ contractility

★ · Dobutamine (1) preferred

· Digoxin

· Dopamine: dose driven

· Preload: Nitroglycerin } vasodilate

· Afterload: Natropresside }

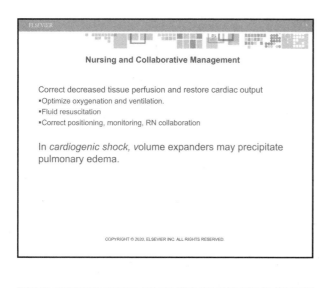

Nursing and Collaborative Management

Correct decreased tissue perfusion and restore cardiac output
- Optimize oxygenation and ventilation.
- Fluid resuscitation
- Correct positioning, monitoring, RN collaboration

In *cardiogenic shock,* volume expanders may precipitate pulmonary edema.

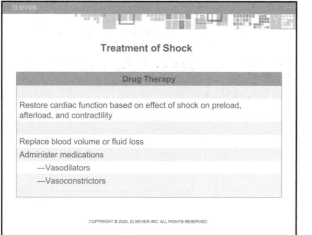

Treatment of Shock

Drug Therapy
Restore cardiac function based on effect of shock on preload, afterload, and contractility
Replace blood volume or fluid loss
Administer medications
—Vasodilators
—Vasoconstrictors

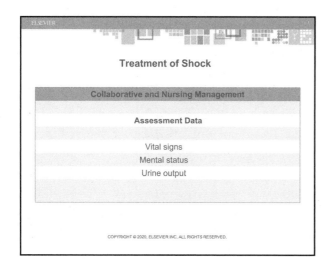

Treatment of Shock

Collaborative and Nursing Management
Assessment Data
Vital signs
Mental status
Urine output

Cardiac tamponade: Becks Triad
JVD, hypotension, muffled ♡ sounds

MAP:

$$\frac{SBP \times (2) Diastolic}{3}$$

Question

A client in shock develops a mean arterial pressure (MAP) of 60 mm Hg and a heart rate of 110 beats per minute. Which prescribed intervention should the nurse implement first?

A. Increase the rate of O_2 flow.

B. Obtain arterial blood gas results.

C. Insert an indwelling urinary catheter.

D. Increase the rate of intravenous (IV) fluids.

Question

A client with a known cardiac history is admitted to the acute care unit with stable angina. At 7:00 a.m., the client had stable vital signs and was on 2 L of oxygen via nasal cannula. At 10:00 a.m., the client reports chest pain of 6 on a scale of 1 to 10, is slightly diaphoretic and pale, has a blood pressure (BP) of 100/52 mm Hg, and has a respiratory rate of 24 breaths/min. Which action should the nurse implement first?

A. Apply 4 L of oxygen as ordered.

B. Administer a fluid bolus of 0.9 normal saline.

C. Administer the prescribed opioid for pain control.

D. Obtain a full set of vital signs, including temperature.

Handwritten notes:

known ♡ hx.

↑O_2 needs to myocardium

If BP not provided, need that assessed first.

Question

A client with burn injuries has lost a significant amount of body fluid. An IV of lactated Ringer's solution is infusing at 200 mL/hour, and the client's urine output for the past 8 hours is 400 mL. Which sign or symptom is the top priority in early distributive shock?

A. A change in BP from 118/60 to 102/68

B. A change in level of consciousness from awake to restless

C. A decrease in O_2 saturation from 98% to 93%

D. A decrease in urine output over 8 hours from 400 to 240 mL

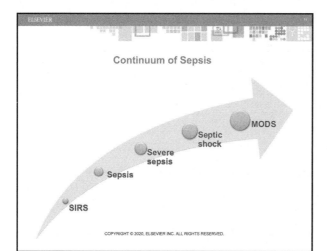

Continuum of Sepsis

MODS

Septic shock

Severe sepsis

Sepsis

SIRS

Sepsis

- Systemic inflammatory response (SIRS) is an assortment of insults, including sepsis, ischemia, infarction, and injury.
- Generalized inflammation occurs in organs remote from the initial insult.
- SIRS usually starts with an infection.
- Septic shock is one component of the SIRS.

- Syndrome starts with an infection that progresses to bacteremia, then sepsis, then severe sepsis, then septic shock, and finally multiple organ dysfunction syndrome (MODS).
- The prognosis for MODS is poor.

Sepsis: Nursing and Collaborative Management

- The most important goal is to prevent the progression of SIRS to MODS.
- The nursing role is attentive data collection and ongoing monitoring to detect early signs of organ dysfunction.
- Collaborative care focuses on:
  ✓ Prevention strategies
  ✓ Early recognition of subtle changes in HR, systolic BP, respiratory rate, oxygen saturation, urinary output, and CNS changes
  ✓ Serum lactate and glucose levels
  ✓ Prevention and treatment of infection
    - Blood culture before antibiotics
    - Broad-spectrum antibiotics within 1 to 3 hours of admission
  ✓ Maintenance of tissue oxygenation
  ✓ Nutritional and metabolic support
  ✓ Support of individual failing organs

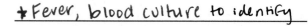

✱ Fever, blood culture to identify pathogen. 2 sets.

· Broad-spectrum ABX before identified.

↑BG. Draw lactate levels (↑)

DIC: Disseminated Intravascular Coagulation

- DIC is a serious disorder of homeostasis resulting from overstimulation of clotting factors followed by anticlotting processes in response to diseases or injury
- Astute ongoing evaluation and assessment is needed.

DIC: Disseminated Intravascular Coagulation

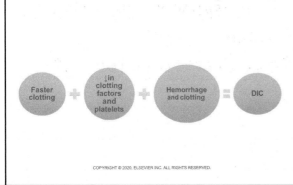

DIC

- DIC may lead to uncontrollable hemorrhage
- Early detection of bleeding, both occult & overt, is the primary goal
- d-dimer assay measures the degree of fibrinolysis (fibrin products in the blood)
- Assess the client for signs of external and internal bleeding
- Be alert for manifestations of the syndrome

Appropriate treatment measures can be challenging and sometimes paradoxic.

- Heparin infusion (early in DIC, when clots are forming)
- Blood, FFP transfusions, and cryoprecipitate

"Oozing of blood"
Notify HCP ★

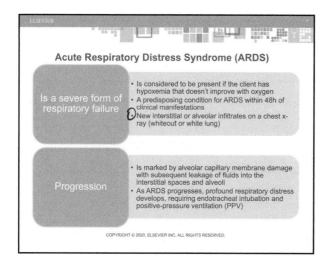

Acute Respiratory Distress Syndrome (ARDS)

Is a severe form of respiratory failure
- Is considered to be present if the client has hypoxemia that doesn't improve with oxygen
- A predisposing condition for ARDS within 48h of clinical manifestations
- New interstitial or alveolar infiltrates on a chest x-ray (whiteout or white lung)

Progression
- Is marked by alveolar capillary membrane damage with subsequent leakage of fluids into the interstitial spaces and alveoli
- As ARDS progresses, profound respiratory distress develops, requiring endotracheal intubation and positive-pressure ventilation (PPV)

ARDS: Nursing Assessment

- Hypoxemia
- Dyspnea
- Scattered crackles
- Increased work of breathing
- Intercostal retractions
- Respiratory acidosis (early)
- Pleural effusions
- Decreased cardiac output
- Cyanosis

A — Pulmonary capillary
Alveolus
B — Interstitium / Pulmonary capillary
C

ARDS: Nursing and Collaborative Management

Overall Goals
- PaO_2 of at least 60 mm Hg
- Adequate lung ventilation to maintain normal pH

Goals for Recovering Patient
- PaO_2 within normal limits for age or baseline values on room air
- SaO_2 >90%
- Patent airway
- Clear lungs on auscultation

Handwritten notes:

O_2 in and CO_2 out both difficult

Respiratory alkalosis turns to acidosis ① ②

CXR white out

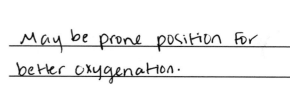

May be prone position for better oxygenation.

Delirium

An **acute state** of confusion and
difficulty concentrating
-Common among elderly,
hospitalized clients
-May indicate an impending change
in condition (i.e., sepsis, urinary
tract infection)

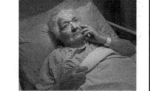

Risk Factors
- Sleep deprivation, advanced age, or
vision and hearing impairment
- Use of opioids and/or corticosteroids
- Drug or alcohol abuse
- UTI, fluid and electrolyte imbalance
- Postoperative (unscheduled surgery),
ICU, or emergent delirium

Delirium: Nursing and Collaborative Management

- Prevention and early recognition (monitor neurological status)
- Protect the client from harm.
- Provide a low-stimulation environment (calm).
- Provide the appropriate level of supervision/surveillance.
- Reorient the client and communicate with simple statements.
- Consider management with neuroleptic drugs (e.g., haloperidol
[Haldol]) as prescribed.
- Encourage family visibility and support.

Question

**A client recovering from ARDS is awake and alert but has residual
fatigue and generalized weakness. The client's current vital signs
are heart rate 83 beats per minute, blood pressure 104/64 mm Hg,
respiratory rate 25 breaths/min, SpO$_2$ is 92% on 2 L/min oxygen
via nasal cannula. Which vital sign finding should the unlicensed
assistive personnel (UAP) immediately report to the nurse?**

A. Heart rate of 83 beats per minute
B. Blood pressure of 104/64 mm Hg
C. Respiratory rate of 25 breaths/minute
D. SpO$_2$ 92% of 2L/min O$_2$ via nasal cannula

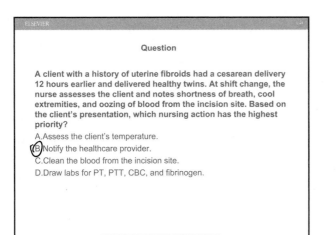

Question

A client is admitted with a 2-day history of cough, fever, and fatigue. The medical history is positive for type I diabetes and recent upper respiratory infection (URI). Vital signs are heart rate 109 beats per minute, blood pressure 102/58 mm Hg, respiratory rate 24 breaths/min, temperature 104°F (40°C), and SpO_2 92% on 2 L oxygen via nasal cannula. Which prescription has the highest priority in this client's care?

A. Initiate large-bore IV access.
B. Draw two sets of blood cultures.
C. Administer the ordered IV antibiotics.
D. Draw serum lactate and glucose levels.

Question

A client with a history of uterine fibroids had a cesarean delivery 12 hours earlier and delivered healthy twins. At shift change, the nurse assesses the client and notes shortness of breath, cool extremities, and oozing of blood from the incision site. Based on the client's presentation, which nursing action has the highest priority?

A. Assess the client's temperature.
B. Notify the healthcare provider.
C. Clean the blood from the incision site.
D. Draw labs for PT, PTT, CBC, and fibrinogen.

Life Support

Cardiac arrest is the most common event requiring CPR.
- **CAB:** *Chest compressions–Airway–Breathing*
  - High-quality chest compressions
  - Push hard and push fast.
  - Adult: 100 to 120 compressions/min

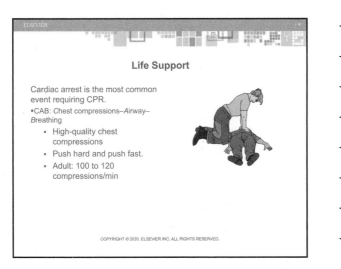

Life Support

In-Hospital Cardiac Arrest
- Initiate CPR with BCLS guidelines.
- Determine unresponsiveness.
- Activate emergency response or cardiac arrest team.
- Call for AED and/or emergency crash cart (do not leave client).
- Initiate compressions.
  - After 30 compressions, open airway with head-tilt-chin lift and ventilate with bag-valve mask (provide 2 breaths, each over 1 second).
  - Maintain compressions-to-breaths ratio of 30:2.
- Once the defibrillator or AED arrives, apply "quick-look" paddles or AED to determine whether defibrillation is necessary; defibrillate as indicated according to hospital policies and procedures.
- Resume CPR.

CPR and Choking Basics:
Neonates and Children Ages 1 to 8

- Indications for CPR in children are different than those for adults.
  - **Neonates and infants:** hypoxia, hypoglycemia, hypothermia, acidosis, hypercoagulability
  - **Children:** respiratory arrest, prolonged hypoxemia secondary to respiratory insult or shock, including septic shock
- Guidelines vary based on age of child.
  - If no response occurs, call a "code," or cardiac arrest, to initiate response of cardiac arrest team.
  - Obtain AED or emergency crash cart with defibrillator.

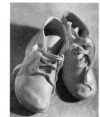

CPR and Choking Basics:
Neonates and Children Ages 1 to 8

- Guidelines vary based on age of child.
  - Check for pulse.
    - Infant aged <1 year: brachial pulse
    - Children aged 1 year to puberty: carotid or femoral
  - Compressions (begin within 10 seconds)
    - *Infants*: Compressions cover 1/3 of anterior/posterior diameter of chest; depth is inches.
    - *Children*: Compressions cover 1/3 of anterior/posterior diameter of chest; depth is 2 inches.
  - Deliver each breath over 1 second.

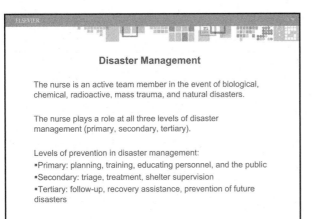

Question

The nurse finds a client slumped in a chair. Place the nurse's actions in order of priority from first to last for this client.

A. Activate the code team and obtain defibrillator. *2*
B. Determine unresponsiveness. *1*
C. Assess the cardiac rhythm using the "quick-look" paddles. *7*
D. Assess for a carotid pulse. *3*
E. Open airway and give two rescue breaths by bag-valve mask. *6*
F. Move the client to a flat position in bed or on the floor. *4*
G. Begin compressions. *5*

Disaster Management

The nurse is an active team member in the event of biological, chemical, radioactive, mass trauma, and natural disasters.

The nurse plays a role at all three levels of disaster management (primary, secondary, tertiary).

Levels of prevention in disaster management:
- Primary: planning, training, educating personnel, and the public
- Secondary: triage, treatment, shelter supervision
- Tertiary: follow-up, recovery assistance, prevention of future disasters

---

Triage

- The goal of triage is to maximize the number of survivors by sorting the injured as treatable and untreatable, using the criteria of potential for survival and availability of resources.
- Color-coded system (in order of priority)
  - *Red*: life-threatening, need immediate intervention
  - *Yellow*: injuries with systemic effects and complications
  - *Green*: minor injuries, no systemic complications
  - *Black*: dying or deceased—catastrophic injuries
- START (**S**imple **T**riage **A**nd **R**apid **T**reatment) method
- Identify the walking wounded; move them to an area where they can be evaluated later.
- Three-step evaluation of others, done one at a time:
  - Assess respirations
  - Assess circulation
  - Assess mental status

B, D, A, C

Question

Four clients arrive in the emergency department after an explosion. In which order should they be assessed? All options must be used.

A. A 70-year-old who is complaining of a pain level of 8/10 from a hand burn *[3]*

B. A 35-year-old with partial and full-thickness burns to the anterior and posterior chest *[1]*

C. A 25-year-old with a superficial burn to the right anterior arm and lateral chest *[4]*

D. A 42-year-old with a partial-thickness burn to the anterior lower extremity and confusion *[2]*

Question

The nurse is assessing clients at the site of a community disaster. Using the color-code system for triage, which client should the nurse tag with a red code?

A. A client with a large head injury that is bleeding, an open chest wound, cyanotic skin, no capillary refill, and agonal respirations

B. A client with bruising and swelling of the right forearm, assorted lacerations to the face and neck, dry skin, normal capillary refill, and a respiratory rate of 18

C. A client with scratches and scrapes to the head and face who is limping and helping other clients at the scene

D. A client with an open wound to the abdomen, and a deformed right femur, pulse 125, delayed capillary refill, respiratory rate 32, who is moaning ✓

Bioterrorism

- Review exposure information, assessment, findings, and treatment for various agents.

- Questions may deal with disasters and bioterrorism as they affect the individual victims, families, and the community.

- Sarin: poison Sarin Gas
- Ricin: poison
  ↓ Symptom management
  ✓ Potentially lethal
  Antidote: atropine sulfate
- Radiation: ARS (lethal) 1 wk
  Acute radiation syndrome

ELSEVIER

Question

The nurse is assigned to receive a client in the emergency department with suspected anthrax exposure predecontamination. Which transmission precautions should be most appropriate for the client? (Select all that apply.)

A. Airborne
B. Contact
C. Aplastic
D. Droplet
E. Standard

ELSEVIER

Question

The emergency department nurse is assessing a client with a vesicular rash as a result of suspected smallpox exposure. Which transmission precautions should be most appropriate for this client? (Select all that apply.)

A. Airborne
B. Contact
C. Aplastic
D. Droplet
E. Standard

ELSEVIER

Question

The nurse is caring for a client in shock of unknown etiology and observes the rhythm on the right on the monitor. Which is the nurse's priority intervention?

A. Check for a carotid pulse.
B. Defibrillate the patient with 360 joules of energy.
C. Administer an intravenous saline bolus.
D. Give two breaths via Ambu® bag.

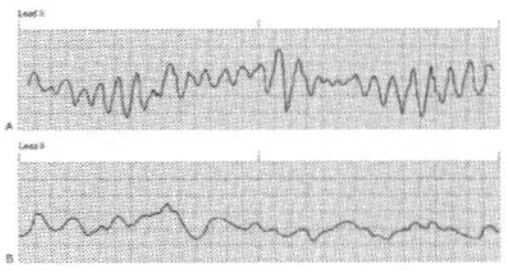

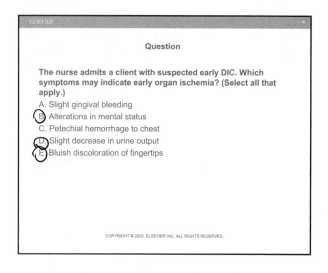

Question

The nurse admits a client with suspected early DIC. Which symptoms may indicate early organ ischemia? (Select all that apply.)

A. Slight gingival bleeding
B. Alterations in mental status
C. Petechial hemorrhage to chest
D. Slight decrease in urine output
E. Bluish discoloration of fingertips

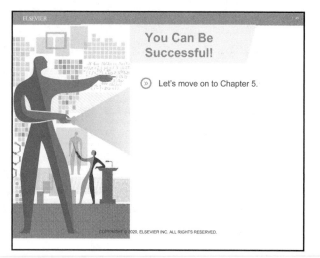

You Can Be Successful!

» Let's move on to Chapter 5.

Oxygenation, Ventilation, Transportation, and Perfusion

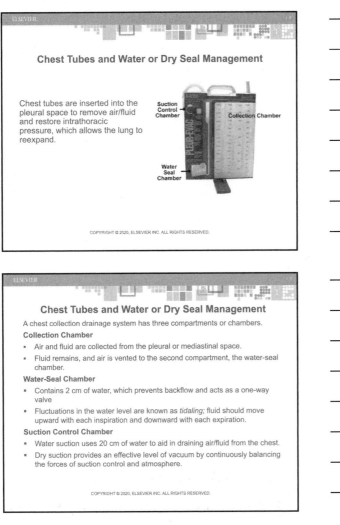

Chest Tubes and Water or Dry Seal Management

Chest tubes are inserted into the pleural space to remove air/fluid and restore intrathoracic pressure, which allows the lung to reexpand.

Suction Control Chamber

Collection Chamber

Water Seal Chamber

Chest Tubes and Water or Dry Seal Management

A chest collection drainage system has three compartments or chambers.

Collection Chamber

- Air and fluid are collected from the pleural or mediastinal space.
- Fluid remains, and air is vented to the second compartment, the water-seal chamber.

Water-Seal Chamber

- Contains 2 cm of water, which prevents backflow and acts as a one-way valve
- Fluctuations in the water level are known as *tidaling;* fluid should move upward with each inspiration and downward with each expiration.

Suction Control Chamber

- Water suction uses 20 cm of water to aid in draining air/fluid from the chest.
- Dry suction provides an effective level of vacuum by continuously balancing the forces of suction control and atmosphere.

Nursing and Collaborative Management

- Check that water level is accurate at 2 cm every shift; add sterile water to chamber if needed.
- Keep unit lower than client's chest.
- Keep unit straight and all tubing loosely coiled below chest level, with all connections tight and taped.
- Monitor the fluid drainage and mark the time of measurement and the fluid level; notify healthcare provider if there is >70 mL/h drainage.
- Monitor respiratory effort and pain levels.
- Assess for tidaling; observe for air bubbling in the water-seal chamber and fluctuations (tidaling).
- Replace the unit when full.
- If chest tube is accidentally dislodged, then:
  - Cover with a dry sterile dressing.
  - If an air leak is noted, tape on three sides.
  - Notify HCP stat.

Ø clamp tubing unless HCP says so

Question

The nurse is precepting a nurse orientee who's caring for a client with a chest tube. The client is 12 hours postoperative from a left partial pneumonectomy. Which assessment will the nurse advise the orientee to immediately report to the healthcare provider? (Select all that apply.)

A. Pain level of 6 out of 10 on the left side
B. Tracheal deviation toward the right side
C. Drainage from the chest tube of 50 mL in the last hour
D. Oxygen saturation of 90% on 2 L/min
E. Vigorous bubbling in the suction chamber

Question

The nurse palpates a crackling sensation around the insertion site of a chest tube in a client who has had thoracic surgery. Which action should the nurse take?

A. Return the client to surgery.

B. Prepare for insertion of a larger chest tube.

C. Increase the water-seal suction pressure.

D. Continue to monitor the insertion site.

Pneumonia

Inflammation of lung tissue, causing consolidation of exudate

Etiology

- Bacterial (gram-negative is the most severe), viral, fungal (rare), or aspiration
- Community-acquired pneumonia (CAP) or hospital-acquired pneumonia (HAP)
- Ventilator-associated pneumonia (VAP)

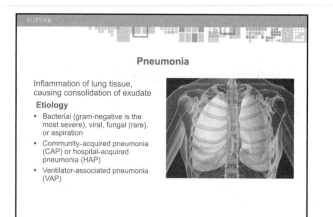

Aspiration pneumonia ↑
risk: muscle weakness, ↓LOC
ex. post stroke.
   · thicken liquid, soft food,
HOB ↑. Tube feeds: check
for residual.

Pneumonia

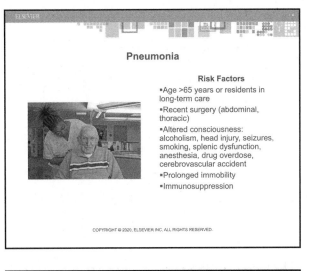

Risk Factors
- Age >65 years or residents in long-term care
- Recent surgery (abdominal, thoracic)
- Altered consciousness: alcoholism, head injury, seizures, smoking, splenic dysfunction, anesthesia, drug overdose, cerebrovascular accident
- Prolonged immobility
- Immunosuppression

Pneumonia

Prevention

- Pneumococcal conjugate vaccine for young children aged >2 years and adults aged ≥65 years
- Pneumococcal polysaccharide (Pneumovac) for all adults aged ≥65 years and children aged ≥2 years at increased risk for pneumonia
- Influenza vaccine yearly

VAP Practice Bundle
- Meticulous hand hygiene
- HOB elevation 30 to 45 degrees
- Oral care per facility protocol
- Suction only as needed with aseptic technique
- Use routine peptic ulcer prophylaxis
- Sedation/weaning protocols
- Early mobilization protocols

Pneumonia

Nursing Assessment
- Tachypnea
- Productive cough
- Pleuritic pain
- Fever of abrupt onset
- Dyspnea
- Increased tactile fremitus
- Mental status changes
- Crackles, decreased breath sounds
- Dullness on percussion
- ABGs indicative of hypoxemia

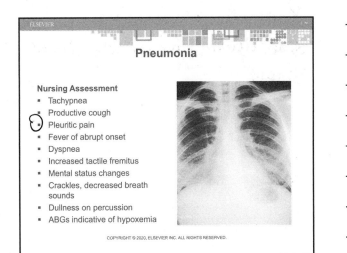

★ pain management

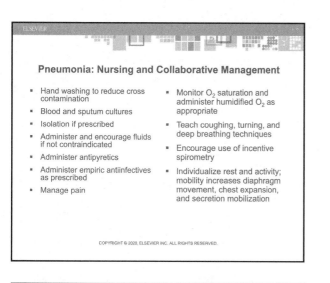

Pneumonia: Nursing and Collaborative Management

- Hand washing to reduce cross contamination
- Blood and sputum cultures
- Isolation if prescribed
- Administer and encourage fluids if not contraindicated
- Administer antipyretics
- Administer empiric antiinfectives as prescribed
- Manage pain

- Monitor O_2 saturation and administer humidified O_2 as appropriate
- Teach coughing, turning, and deep breathing techniques
- Encourage use of incentive spirometry
- Individualize rest and activity; mobility increases diaphragm movement, chest expansion, and secretion mobilization

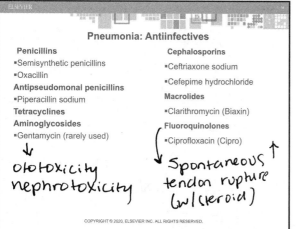

Pneumonia: Antiinfectives

Penicillins
- Semisynthetic penicillins
- Oxacillin

Antipseudomonal penicillins
- Piperacillin sodium

Tetracyclines

Aminoglycosides
- Gentamycin (rarely used)

↓
ototoxicity
nephrotoxicity

Cephalosporins
- Ceftriaxone sodium
- Cefepime hydrochloride

Macrolides
- Clarithromycin (Biaxin)

Fluoroquinolones
- Ciprofloxacin (Cipro)

↓ Spontaneous ↑ tendon rupture (w/ steroid)

Question

A client who is 1 day postoperative after a left pneumonectomy is lying on his right side with the head of bed (HOB) elevated 10 degrees. The nurse assesses his respiratory rate at 32 breaths/min. What action should the nurse take first?

A. Elevate the HOB.
B. Assist the client into the supine position.
C. Measure the client's O_2 saturation.
D. Administer intravenous (IV) PRN morphine.

---

tetracyclines: ∅ pregnancy + children (discolors teeth)
∅ take w/ milk or antacids.
· photosensitivity
Macrolides → 1 wk before antidepressants.

Reposition: Operative side down. Risk: mediastinal shift.

ELSEVIER

Question

The nurse is orienting a graduate nurse (GN) caring for a client dependent on a ventilator. Which action by the GN demonstrates understanding of ventilator-associated pneumonia (VAP) care? (Select all that apply.)

A. Administers a proton pump inhibitor as prescribed
B. Rinses client's oral cavity with chlorhexidine every 2 hours
C. Elevates the HOB 60 degrees
D. Implements spontaneous breathing trial
E. Performs hand hygiene before and after care

ø spontaneous

ELSEVIER

Chronic Airflow Limitation (CAL)

Asthma
- Reversible disease

Chronic obstructive pulmonary disease (COPD)
- Chronic progressive disease
  - Emphysema
  - Chronic bronchitis

ELSEVIER

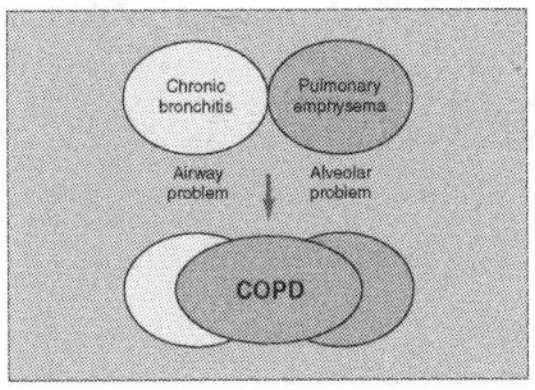

Etiology and Prescription Factors

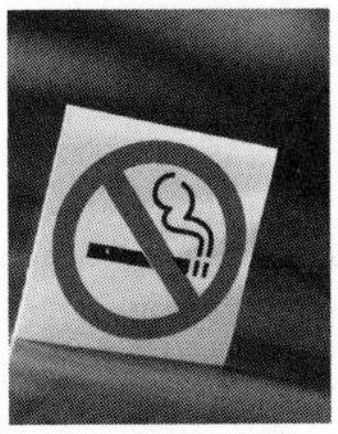

- Cigarette smoking
- Environmental exposure
- Occupational exposure
- Genetic predisposition

90% O2 sat target

Cor pulmonale: RHF
R HF: liver monitoring for
cirrhosis

Air trapping.
· Normal O2, may retain
CO2. Goal: ↓ work of
breathing.

Chronic Bronchitis: Pathophysiology

- Chronic cough with sputum production on a daily basis for a minimum of 3 months/year
- Chronic hypoxemia/cor pulmonale
- Increased mucus production
- Increased bronchial wall thickness (obstructs air flow)
- Exacerbations usually due to infection
- Increased CO_2 retention/acidemia
- Reduced responsiveness of respiratory center to hypoxemic stimuli

Emphysema

- Abnormal enlargement of the air spaces distal to the terminal alveolar walls
- Increased dyspnea/work of breathing
  - Reduced gas exchange surface area
  - Increased air trapping (increased anterior-posterior diameter)
  - Decreased capillary network
  - Increased work/increased O_2 consumption

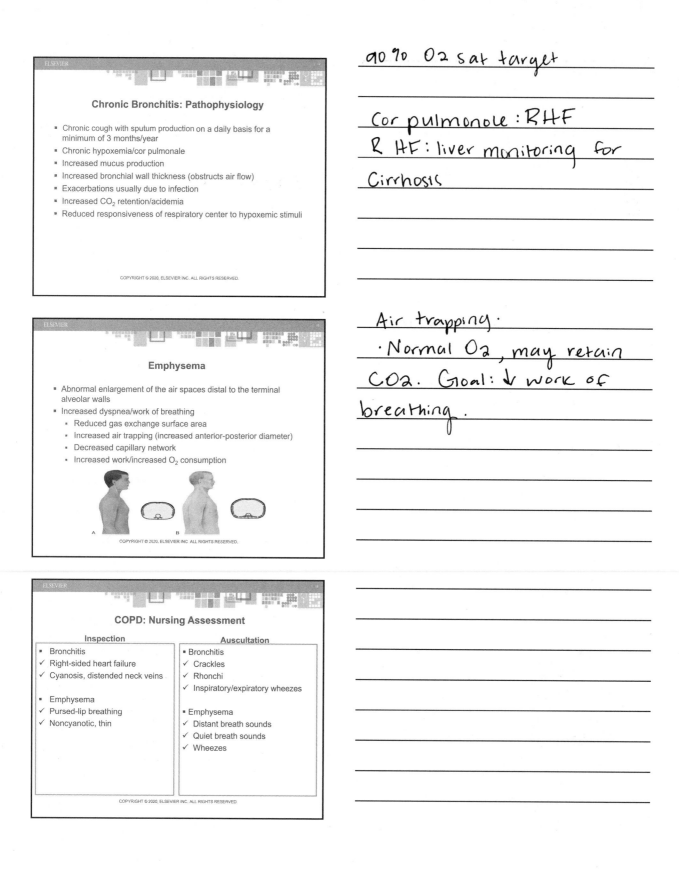

COPD: Nursing Assessment

Inspection	Auscultation
▪ Bronchitis	▪ Bronchitis
✓ Right-sided heart failure	✓ Crackles
✓ Cyanosis, distended neck veins	✓ Rhonchi
	✓ Inspiratory/expiratory wheezes
▪ Emphysema	
✓ Pursed-lip breathing	▪ Emphysema
✓ Noncyanotic, thin	✓ Distant breath sounds
	✓ Quiet breath sounds
	✓ Wheezes

COPD: Nursing and Collaborative Management

Keep SaO_2 to >90% during rest, sleep, and exertion, or the PaO_2 >60 mm Hg.
Long-term continuous O_2 therapy (LTOT) more than 15 hours per day:
▪Increases survival, exercise tolerance, and improved mental status in clients with hypoxemia
▪Maintain infection control techniques
Monitor for signs and symptoms (S/S) of fluid overload.
Baseline ABGs for CO_2 retainers
Teach the client pursed-lip breathing.
Orthopneic position
✖ Nutrition consult
Acute exacerbation
  management

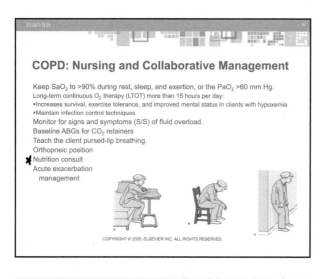

Handwritten note (right margin): high calorie-mechanical soft diet.

Question

A client with pneumonia has impending respiratory failure. Which set of ABG values demonstrate acute respiratory failure?

A. pH–7.30 PCO_2–52 PO_2–56 HCO_3–26
B. pH–7.35 PCO_2–44 PO_2–86 HCO_3–28
C. pH–7.35 PCO_2–62 PO_2–66 HCO_3–31
D. pH–7.30 PCO_2–39 PO_2–88 HCO_3–22

(Answer A is circled)

Reactive Airway Disease

Asthma
  Reversible inflammatory disorder of the airways characterized by an exaggerated bronchoconstrictor response to a wide variety of stimuli
  ▪ Allergens
  ▪ Environmental irritants
  ▪ Cold air
  ▪ Exercise
  ▪ Beta-blockers
  ▪ Respiratory infection
  ▪ Emotional stress
  ▪ Reflux esophagitis

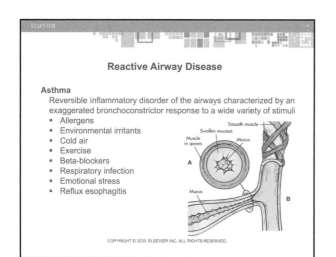

Drug Therapy for Asthma and COPD

- Asthma Medication Goals
  - Quick-relief medications
  - Long-term control medications

- COPD Medication Goals
  - Reduce exacerbations.
  - Long-acting beta-agonists
  - Intercostal space inhaled corticosteroids internal carotid stenosis (ICS)

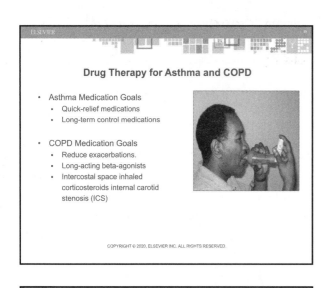

Drug Therapy for Asthma and COPD

Bronchodilators
- Short-acting inhaled β_2-adrenergic agonists
- Long-acting inhaled β_2-adrenergic agonists
- Long-acting oral β_2-adrenergic agonists
- Anticholinergics (inhaled)
  - Ipratropium
  - Aclidinium bromide

Drug Therapy for Asthma and COPD

- **β_2-Adrenergic Agonists**

Inhaled: Short Acting
- Metaproterenol: nebulizer, oral tablets, elixir, metered-dose inhaler (MDI)
- Salbutamol sulfate: nebulizer, MDI, oral tablets
- Levalbuterol: nebulizer, MDI
- Terbutaline: oral tablets, nebulizer, subcutaneous, MDI
- Bitolterol: MDI, nebulizer

- **Inhaled: Long Acting**
  - Salmeterol xinafoate: dry powder inhaler (DPI)
  - Formoterol fumarate: DPI
- **Immediate Acting**
  - Epinephrine hydrochloride: (1:1000) subcutaneous
- **Corticosteroids**

Handwritten notes:

Side effects:
Tachycardia
Urinary retention

Rinse mouth after using an inhaler w/ corticosteroids

ELSEVIER

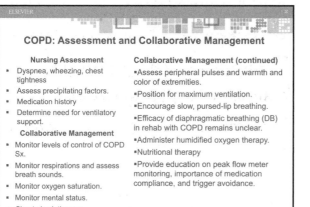

COPD: Assessment and Collaborative Management

Nursing Assessment

- Dyspnea, wheezing, chest tightness
- Assess precipitating factors.
- Medication history
- Determine need for ventilatory support.

Collaborative Management

- Monitor levels of control of COPD Sx.
- Monitor respirations and assess breath sounds.
- Monitor oxygen saturation.
- Monitor mental status.
- Chest physiotherapy

Collaborative Management (continued)

- Assess peripheral pulses and warmth and color of extremities.
- Position for maximum ventilation.
- Encourage slow, pursed-lip breathing.
- Efficacy of diaphragmatic breathing (DB) in rehab with COPD remains unclear.
- Administer humidified oxygen therapy.
- Nutritional therapy
- Provide education on peak flow meter monitoring, importance of medication compliance, and trigger avoidance.

Anaphylaxis: provide reassurance, ↓ anxiety

ELSEVIER

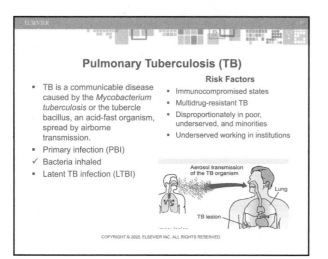

Pulmonary Tuberculosis (TB)

- TB is a communicable disease caused by the *Mycobacterium tuberculosis* or the tubercle bacillus, an acid-fast organism, spread by airborne transmission.
- Primary infection (PBI)
- ✓ Bacteria inhaled
- Latent TB infection (LTBI)

Risk Factors

- Immunocompromised states
- Multidrug-resistant TB
- Disproportionately in poor, underserved, and minorities
- Underserved working in institutions

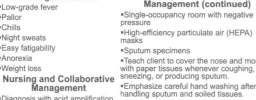

Aerosol transmission of the TB organism
Lung
TB lesion

COPYRIGHT © 2020, ELSEVIER INC. ALL RIGHTS RESERVED.

ELSEVIER

Nursing Assessment and Collaborative Management

Nursing Assessment

- Low-grade fever
- Pallor
- Chills
- Night sweats
- Easy fatigability
- Anorexia
- Weight loss

Nursing and Collaborative Management

- Diagnosis with acid amplification test (NAAT), QuantiFERON-TB or purified protein derivative (PPD) (Mantoux test)
- Notify public health department.
- Airborne precautions isolation

Nursing and Collaborative Management (continued)

- Single-occupancy room with negative pressure
- High-efficiency particulate air (HEPA) masks
- Sputum specimens
- Teach client to cover the nose and mouth with paper tissues whenever coughing, sneezing, or producing sputum.
- Emphasize careful hand washing after handling sputum and soiled tissues.
- If client needs to be out of the negative-pressure room, he or she must wear a standard isolation mask to prevent exposure to others.

COPYRIGHT © 2020, ELSEVIER INC. ALL RIGHTS RESERVED.

TB Drugs and Side Effects

First-Line Drugs

First-line drugs are bacteriocidal against rapidly dividing cells and/or against semidormant bacteria.

- **Isoniazid (INH):** clinical hepatitis, fulminant hepatitis, peripheral neurotoxicity
- **Rifampin (Rifadin, Rofact):** cutaneous reactions, GI disturbance (nausea, anorexia, abdominal pain), flulike syndrome, hepatotoxicity, immunological reactions, orange discoloration of bodily fluids (sputum, urine, sweat, tears)
- **Ethambutol hydrochloride (Etibi):** retrobulbar neuritis (decreased red-green color discrimination), skin rash
- **Rifabutin (Mycobutin):** hematologic toxicity, GI symptoms, polyarthralgias, pseudojaundice, orange discoloration of bodily fluids
- **Pyrazinamide (PZA):** hepatotoxicity, GI symptoms (nausea, vomiting), polyarthralgias, skin rash, hyperuricemia, dermatitis

Managing Active TB

- 8 weeks with INH, Rifampin, Ethamutol, and PZA
- Followed by 18 weeks of INH and Rifampin

Question

The nurse is preparing to administer a purified protein derivative (PPD) test to a client who is entering nursing school. Which action is the nurse's highest priority?

A. Prepare 0.1-mL solution for tuberculin syringe.

B. Assess the skin condition on the forearm.

C. Teach the client about positive findings.

D. Inquire about bacillus Calmette-Guérin (BCG) vaccine history.

Pulmonary Embolus

Any substance can cause an embolism. Typically, a blood clot enters the venous circulation and lodges in the pulmonary vasculature.

Risk Factors for VTE Leading to PE
- Prolonged immobility
- Central venous catheters
- Surgery in last 3 months
- Obesity
- Malignancy
- Clotting disorders
- History of thromboembolism
- Smoking, BCP, pregnancy
- Heart failure

Handwritten notes:

- INH: liver toxicity, ∅ alcohol or deterrent. ↑ Dilantin levels
- Rifampin: orange-tinged ↑ digoxin, hypoglycemics
- Ethambutol: 6 mo vision screening

Pulmonary Embolus: Signs and Symptoms

- Dyspnea, tachypnea, tachycardia
- Sharp, stabbing chest pain
- Cough, hemoptysis
- Crackles, pleural friction rub
- $\downarrow SO_2$ saturation, respiratory alkalosis, then respiratory acidosis
- Pleural friction rub
- S_3 or S_4 heart sound
- Feeling of impending doom
- Low-grade fever
- Hemoptysis
- Hypoxemia

- Elevated D-dimer level
- Diagnosed by findings: spiral CT, transesophageal echocardiography (TEE), V/Q scan

---

PE: Nursing and Collaborative Management

Prevention
- Range-of-motion exercises
- Ambulate and turn.
- Avoid popliteal pressure.
- Use antiembolism and pneumatic compression stockings.
- Assess peripheral circulation.
- Administer prescribed prophylactic anticoagulant and antiplatelet drugs.
- Teach client and family about precautions.
- Encourage client to stop smoking and to exercise.

Acute Management
- Oxygen therapy
- Monitor ABG and pulse oximetry.
- Check vital signs, lung sounds, and cardiac status.
- Embolectomy
- Inferior vena cava filtration with placement of a vena cava filter

---

PE: Nursing and Collaborative Management
High-Risk Medications

Anticoagulants are used to prevent embolus enlargement and the formation of new clots; use with caution with active bleeding, stroke, and recent trauma.

Warfarin (Coumadin) should be initiated within the first 3 days of heparinization and is continued for 3 to 6 months post-PE.

Low-molecular-weight heparin is usually used unless the PE is massive or occurs with hemodynamic instability.

Alteplase (Activase, Cathflo), fibrinolytic drugs

- Therapeutic aPTT values usually range from 1.5 to 2.5 times.

IV heparin for more severe cases

Both **heparin** and fibrinolytic drugs are high-alert drugs.

LVHF: S_3

S_4 may occur after MI

Hematologic Problems:
Anemia and Its Many Causes

- ↓ Erythrocyte production
- ↓ Hemoglobin synthesis
- Iron deficiency
- Defective DNA synthesis
- B_{12} and folic acid deficiency
- ↓ Number of erythrocyte precursors
- Chronic diseases or disorders
- Chemotherapy
- Blood loss
- Blood vessel rupture

- Chronic gastritis
- Trauma
- Menorrhagia
- Hemorrhoids

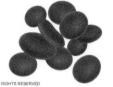

Anemia

Nursing Assessment

- Pallor, fatigue
- Exercise intolerance
- Tachycardia, dyspnea
- Complete blood count
- Assess for risk factors.
- Diet low in iron, vitamin B_{12} deficiency, history of bleeding, medications taken
- Hgb < 10 g/dL (100 mmol/L), Hct <36%, RBC <4×10^{12}/L

Nursing and Collaborative Management

- Treatment of underlying pathology
- Administer blood products as prescribed.
- Encourage diet high in iron-rich foods, folic acid, vitamin B_{12}, vitamin B_6, amino acids, and vitamin C.
- Give parenteral iron via Z-track technique.

Question

The charge nurse is planning client assignments for the unit. The collaborative care team consists of a registered nurse (RN), a practical nurse (PN), and an unlicensed assistive personnel (UAP). Which client(s) should be assigned to the RN? (Select all that apply.)

A. A client awaiting a blood transfusion for gastrointestinal bleeding with an Hgb 7.0 mg/dL (70g/L)

B. A client with pernicious anemia who is awaiting vitamin B_{12} injection

C. A client with resolving sickle cell crisis awaiting IV fluid conversion to saline lock

D. A client with a pressure ulcer who has been prescribed negative pressure wound (vacuum-assisted closure [VAC]) care

E. A client who received two blood transfusions yesterday and is awaiting morning care

---

Diet? Meds?

Blood Transfusions

Blood Groups and Types
- ABO system includes A, B, O, and AB blood types.
- Rh factor is an antigenic substance in the erythrocytes.
- If blood is mismatched during transfusion, a transfusion reaction occurs.
  - Transfusion reaction is an antigen-antibody reaction.
  - It can range from a mild response to severe anaphylactic shock.

Types of Reactions
Acute hemolytic, febrile, nonhemolytic (most common), mild allergic, anaphylactic, delayed hemolytic

Nursing and Collaborative Management
- Perform assessment before, during, and after, including the IV site.
- Determine two identifiers.
- Confirm informed consent.
- Identify the compatibility
- Initiate a transfusion slowly, then maintain the infusion rate.

Types of Blood Products

- RBCs
  - Packed RBCs
  - Autologous RBCs
  - Washed RBCs
  - Frozen RBCs
  - Leukocyte-poor RBCs
  - Young
- Other cellular components
  - Platelets
  - Granulocytes
- Plasma components
  - Fresh frozen plasma (FFP)
  - Cryoprecipitate

Question

A client who is receiving a transfusion of packed red blood cells has an inflamed IV site. Which action should the nurse take?

A. Double-check the blood type of the transfusing unit of blood with another nurse

B. Discontinue the transfusion and send the remaining blood and tubing to the lab

C. Immediately start a new IV at another site and resume the transfusion at the new site

D. Continue to monitor the site for signs of infection and notify the healthcare provider

Hypertension (HTN)

Persistent BP elevation >140/90 mm Hg

Risk Factors

- Nonmodifiable: family history, gender, age, ethnicity
- Modifiable: use of alcohol, tobacco, caffeine; sedentary lifestyle; obesity

Medications

- Diuretics, antihypertensives, ACE inhibitors, calcium channel blockers

HTN Education

- The #1 cause of stroke (CVA, brain attack) is nonadherence to HTN medications.

Coronary Artery Disease (CAD)

CAD is one of the leading causes of morbidity and mortality in the United States and Canada.

CAD results in ischemia and infarction of myocardial tissue.

LAD (left anterior descending artery) is most commonly affected.

Highly sensitive CRP (hsCRP)

Prevalent Etiologies of CAD
- Atherosclerosis: partially or completely blocked coronary arteries
- Coronary vasospasm
- Microvascular angina

Reduction of Risk Factors
- Smoking cessation
- Weight loss–DASH
- Lowering cholesterol levels
- Glycemic control
- Stress reduction
- Medication compliance
- ↑ Activity/exercise

Cholesterol-Lowering Drugs

May be initiated if diet modification is unsuccessful
- Atorvastatin (Lipitor)
- Lovastatin (Mevacor)
- Pravastatin (Pravachol)
- Rosuvastatin (Crestor)
- Simvastatin (Zocor)
- Ezetemibe (Ezetrol)
- Gemfibrozil (Lopid)
- Niacin (nicotinic acid)

*Rhabdomyolysis: medical emergency

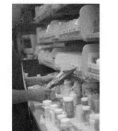

Clonadine: BP emergency
CNS med: body relaxation
· Rebound HTN

Proprandol: works on whole body

"-Statins": muscle breakdown risk

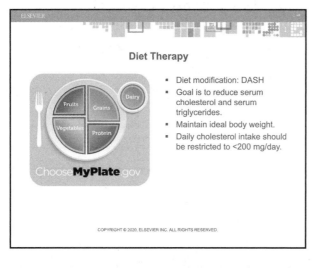

Diet Therapy

- Diet modification: DASH
- Goal is to reduce serum cholesterol and serum triglycerides.
- Maintain ideal body weight.
- Daily cholesterol intake should be restricted to <200 mg/day.

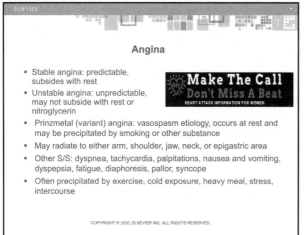

Angina

- Stable angina: predictable, subsides with rest
- Unstable angina: unpredictable, may not subside with rest or nitroglycerin
- Prinzmetal (variant) angina: vasospasm etiology, occurs at rest and may be precipitated by smoking or other substance
- May radiate to either arm, shoulder, jaw, neck, or epigastric area
- Other S/S: dyspnea, tachycardia, palpitations, nausea and vomiting, dyspepsia, fatigue, diaphoresis, pallor, syncope
- Often precipitated by exercise, cold exposure, heavy meal, stress, intercourse

Make The Call
Don't Miss A Beat
HEART ATTACK INFORMATION FOR WOMEN

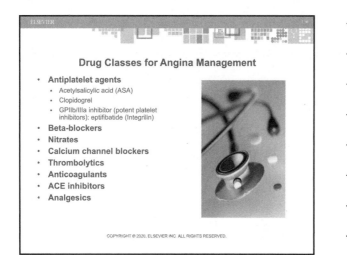

Drug Classes for Angina Management

- **Antiplatelet agents**
  - Acetylsalicylic acid (ASA)
  - Clopidogrel
  - GPIIb/IIIa inhibitor (potent platelet inhibitors): eptifibatide (Integrilin)
- **Beta-blockers**
- **Nitrates**
- **Calcium channel blockers**
- **Thrombolytics**
- **Anticoagulants**
- **ACE inhibitors**
- **Analgesics**

Nitro ∅ ED meds in 48 hrs.
→ severe headache

O₂ based on pt. need

Drug Therapy

Oxygen

Administer oxygen and titrate as appropriate to assist in oxygenating myocardial tissue, especially in those who are hypoxic, those in respiratory distress, or those at high risk.

Nitroglycerin

- Dilates the coronary arteries
- ↑ Blood flow to the damaged area of myocardium

Dose

- 0.4 mg/tablet
- 1 tab sublingual every 5 minutes × 3 doses

Nitrostat
(Nitroglycerin Tablets,USP)
0.4 mg (1/150 gr)
℞ only
100 SUBLINGUAL TABLETS
PARKE-DAVIS

Drug Therapy

Morphine Sulfate	Analgesic; ↓ anxiety; ↓ tachypnea; relaxes bronchial smooth muscle; improves gas exchange
Beta-Blockers	↓ Heart rate; ↓workload of heart; ↓ oxygen demand of myocardium
Calcium Channel Blockers	↓ Conduction through AV node; slow heart rate; ↓ oxygen demand by myocardium
Thrombolytic Therapy (within protocol guidelines)	Useful when infarction is diagnosed early; streptokinase and tPA; administered IV Most effective if given within 6 hours of onset of chest pain; heparin therapy will usually follow thrombolytic therapy

Medical Interventions

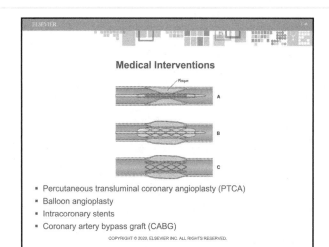

- Percutaneous transluminal coronary angioplasty (PTCA)
- Balloon angioplasty
- Intracoronary stents
- Coronary artery bypass graft (CABG)

Acute Myocardial Infarction (MI)

- Destruction of myocardial tissue due to lack of blood and oxygen supply
- Begins with occlusion of the coronary artery
- Ischemia, injury, infarction
- ST-elevation MI (STEMI) (traditional MI)
- Non-STEMI (common in women)

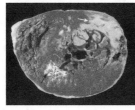

Acute Myocardial Infarction (MI)

Ischemia
- Results from reduced blood flow and oxygen to the coronary arteries
- If not reversed, then injury occurs.
- Ischemia lasting 20 minutes or more is sufficient to produce irreversible tissue damage.
- T-wave inversion on ECG

Injury
- Prolonged interruption of oxygen supply and nutrients
- Cells are still salvageable.
- ST elevation

Infarction
- Tissue necrosis and death
- Irreversible damage
- Scar tissue has no electrical stimulation or contractility.
- Within 24 hours of infarction the healing process begins.
- Pathological Q waves

Myocardial Infarction

Complications

As many as 90% of clients suffer complications, including the following:
- Dysrhythmias
- Cardiac failure
- Cardiogenic shock
- Thromboembolism
- Ventricular rupture

Signs and Symptoms

Pain
- Sudden onset; severity increases
- May persist for hours or days; not relieved by rest or nitroglycerin
- Heavy/constrictive
- Located behind the sternum
- May radiate to arms, back, neck, or jaw

Cool and clammy skin

Rapid, irregular, feeble pulse

· Cardiogenic shock: LV damage

Atypical Symptoms

Women
- Discomfort rather than pain
- Shortness of breath
- Extreme fatigue

Clients With Diabetes
- Asymptomatic
- Neuropathy
- Dyspnea

Elderly Clients
- Confusion/delirium
- Dizziness
- Shortness of breath

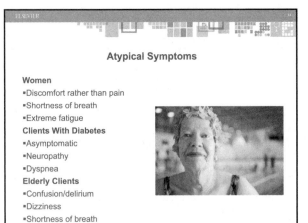

Medical Diagnosis

ECG (12-lead)

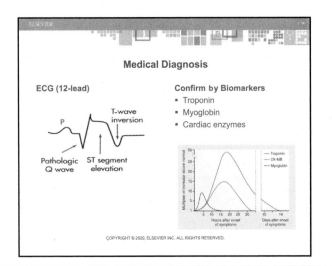

P
T-wave inversion
Pathologic Q wave
ST segment elevation

Confirm by Biomarkers
- Troponin
- Myoglobin
- Cardiac enzymes

Cardiac Lab Tests

Troponin
- Found only in cardiac muscle
- May present as early as 1 hour after injury
- Peaks within 24 hours
- Returns to normal in 5 to 14 days

Myoglobin
- Released 1 hour after an acute myocardial infarction
- Rises before creatine kinase-MB levels
- Returns to normal within 24 hours

Treatment: Preserve Myocardial Tissue

Overall goal is to preserve myocardial tissue within 90 minutes of arrival to the healthcare facility with the following:

- Drug therapy
  - Oxygen
  - Nitroglycerin
  - Beta-blockers
  - Morphine
- Thrombolytic therapy via catherization

- Percutaneous coronary intervention and stents within 90 minutes of presentation for care
- If PCI unavailable, risk versus benefit of intravenous thrombolytic therapy is completed
- Coronary artery bypass graft
- Severe coronary artery disease detected
- Can be emergent or elective

Heart Failure

Etiology

- CAD, prior MI
- Chronic HTN
- Cardiomyopathy
  - Dilated, idiopathic
- Hyperthyroidism
- Diabetes
- Valvular and congenital heart disease
- Pulmonary diseases

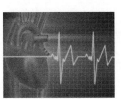

Heart Failure

Left-Sided Heart Failure

Causes: LV infarct, cardiomyopathy, hypertension

Symptoms: dyspnea, cough, orthopnea, pulmonary edema, paroxysmal nocturnal dyspnea

Signs: S3 gallop, tachycardia, inspiratory rales

Laboratory findings: ABGs reveal hypoxemia, CXR shows pulmonary edema or pleural effusions, ↑B-type natriuretic peptide (BNP) >500 ng/mL

Right-Sided Heart Failure

Causes: LHF, RV infarct, pulmonary or tricuspid valve disease, pulmonary HTN, COPD, PE

Symptoms: Systemic congestion, dyspnea on exertion, fatigue, weight gain, fluid retention

Signs: ↑ central venous pressure (CVP), jugular venous distention (JVD) >3 to 4 cm, hepatomegaly, ascites, peripheral or sacral edema, and pleural and pericardial effusions

Block RAAS system

Right Heart Failure Laboratory Tests

Sodium and Volume Homeostasis

As cardiac output decreases, renal perfusion decreases, activating the Renin-Angiotensin-Aldosterone System (RAAS), causing fluid retention.

Laboratory Tests

- Liver function shows hepatic congestion.
- Increased liver enzymes, increased PT and INR
- Hyponatremia (fluid restriction only if Na^+ is <132 mEq/L)
- Increased BUN/creatinine = decreased renal perfusion

Pharmacological Management

- Angiotensin-converting enzyme (ACE) inhibitors
- Diuretics
- Inotropes
- Phosphodiesterase inhibitors
- Natriuretic peptides
- Beta-blockers
- Angiotensin II receptor blockers
- Vasodilators
- Dopamine agonist
- Anticoagulants/antiplatelets/aspirin

Nursing and Collaborative Management

- Administer oxygen as prescribed.
- Reposition and perform coughing, deep-breathing exercises every 2 hours.
- Limit sodium intake.
- Fluid restriction only if Na+ <132 mmol/L (mEq/L)
- Avoid excessive fluids.
- Avoid alcohol—depresses myocardial contractility.
- With CAD, low cholesterol, low fat, low Na+

Educate on signs of worsening condition such as weight gain 1.36 kg (3 lb) weekly or 0.45 to 0.9 kg (1–2 lb) overnight; increasing DOE, orthopnea, or PND.

Regular exercise is strongly encouraged—improves function of skeletal muscle more than changes in myocardial function.

Question

The nurse is administering 0900 medications to three clients on a telemetry unit when the UAP reports that another client is complaining of a sudden onset of substernal discomfort. What action should the nurse take?

A. Ask the UAP to obtain the client's vital signs
B. Assess the client's discomfort
C. Advise the client to rest in bed
D. Observe the client's ECG pattern

Question

A client a history of coronary heart disease was admitted to the acute care unit 2 days ago for management of angina. During the assessment, the client states, "I feel like I have indigestion." In which order should the nurse implement care? (Arrange from first action to last.)

A. Notify the rapid response team.
B. Administer PRN nitroglycerin prescription.
C. Check the pulse, respirations, blood pressure, and oxygen saturation.
D. Document assessment in the electronic medical record.
E. Provide 2 L of oxygen via nasal cannula.

C E B A D

Question

For which dysrhythmia should the nurse implement defibrillation? (Select all that apply.)

A. Asystole
B. Pulseless electrical activity
C. Ventricular fibrillation
D. Pulseless ventricular tachycardia
E. Ventricular tachycardia
F. Atrial fibrillation

Question

The nurse is caring for a client when the client suddenly becomes unconscious. The nurse identifies the following rhythm on the monitor. Which action is the highest priority?

A. Check for a carotid pulse
B. Begin chest compressions
C. Administer epinephrine 1:10,000 IV
D. Initiate bag-valve mask ventilations

Dysrhythmias: Interpretation and Management

Standard ECG uses 12 leads
- Provides best overall evaluation

Telemetry
- Usually 3 leads show one view of the heart.

Holter monitor
- Usually worn for 24-hour continuous reading

- Client may be asymptomatic until cardiac output is altered.
- Client may complain of palpitations, syncope, pain, dyspnea, and diaphoresis.
- Changes in pulse rate/rhythm and ECG will be seen.
- Always treat the client and **NOT** the monitor!

QT: 0.44 sec

Electrocardiogram (ECG)

P wave
- Atrial depolarization

QRS complex
- Ventricular depolarization
- Normal <0.11 second

ST segment
- Early ventricular repolarization

T wave
- Ventricular repolarization

PR interval
- Time for impulse to travel through SA node
- Normal: 0.12 to 0.2 second

R-R interval
- Measure regularity of heartbeat

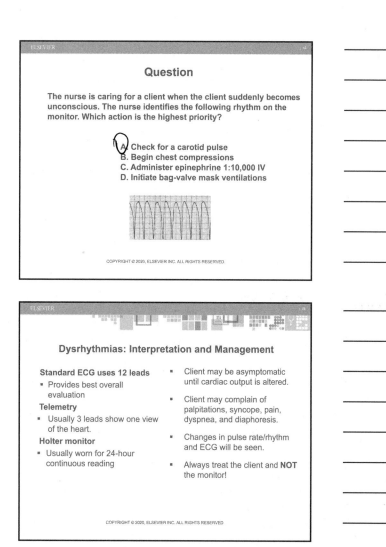

Atrial Dysrhythmias

A-fib (atrial fibrillation)
- Chaotic activity in the AV node
- No true P waves visible
- Irregular R-R intervals
- Risk for CVA
- Anticoagulant therapy is necessary

Atrial Flutter
- Sawtoothed waveform (F waves)
- Regular/irregular R-R interval
- Fluttering in chest
- Ventricular rhythm regular

Cardioversion may be used for either.
Focus is on rate control.
If onset is >48 hours, then TEE is required.
Always ensure sedation prior to cardioversion.

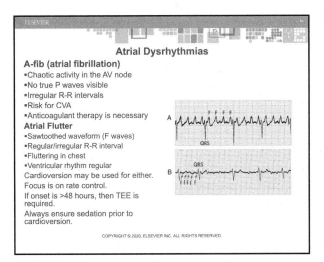

Ventricular Dysrhythmias

V-tach (ventricular tachycardia)
- Wide, bizarre QRS complex
- Assess whether client has a pulse.
- Is cardiac output impaired?
- Prepare for synchronized cardioversion.
- Administer antiarrhythmic drugs.

V-fib (ventricular fibrillation)
- Cardiac emergency
- No cardiac output
- Start cardiopulmonary resuscitation (CPR).
- Defibrillate as quickly as possible.
- Administer antiarrhythmic drugs.

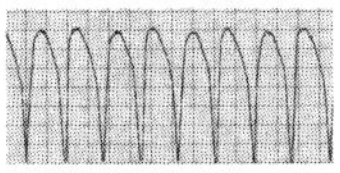

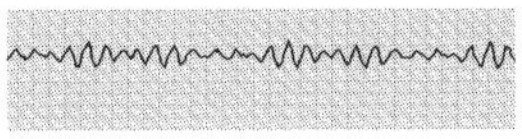

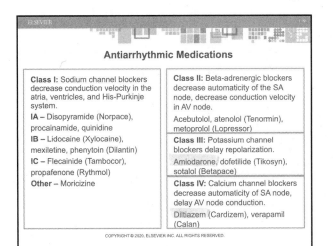

Antiarrhythmic Medications

Class I: Sodium channel blockers decrease conduction velocity in the atria, ventricles, and His-Purkinje system. **IA** – Disopyramide (Norpace), procainamide, quinidine **IB** – Lidocaine (Xylocaine), mexiletine, phenytoin (Dilantin) **IC** – Flecainide (Tambocor), propafenone (Rythmol) **Other** – Moricizine	**Class II:** Beta-adrenergic blockers decrease automaticity of the SA node, decrease conduction velocity in AV node. Acebutolol, atenolol (Tenormin), metoprolol (Lopressor)
	Class III: Potassium channel blockers delay repolarization. Amiodarone, dofetilide (Tikosyn), sotalol (Betapace)
	Class IV: Calcium channel blockers decrease automaticity of SA node, delay AV node conduction. Diltiazem (Cardizem), verapamil (Calan)

Handwritten notes:

- Atrial kick: to fill ventricles for optimal output (1/3)
- Sedation before cardioversion

Diltiazem: A-fib — slows conduction. Can convert rhythm

Question

An older client with a history of hypertension, heart failure, and sleep apnea is admitted to the acute care unit. Which finding(s) should relate most directly to a diagnosis of acute decompensated heart failure? (Select all that apply.)

A. Respiratory rate of 25 breaths/min
B. Orthopnea
C. S3 heart sound
D. Dry, nonproductive cough
E. Heart rate of 69 and irregular

Inflammatory Heart Disease

Endocarditis

- **Signs/symptoms:** fever, positive blood cultures, murmur, hemorrhages, HF symptoms, often with IV drug abuse
- Infective endocarditis can lead to damaged heart valves.
- Assess for right- or left-sided heart failure.
- Administer IV antibiotics for 4 to 6 weeks.
- Maintain balance of rest and physical activity.
- Surgical treatment for valvular damage.
- Teach clients to request prophylactic antibiotics for every invasive procedure (dental included).

Pericarditis

- **Signs/symptoms:** pain—hurts more with deep breath or supine, pericardial friction rub
- Monitor for ST-segment elevation.
- Monitor hemodynamic status.
- Facilitate a leaning-over position and NSAIDs for pain control measures.

Valvular Heart Disease

Valves may be unable to:
- Fully open (stenosis)
- Fully close (insufficiency or regurgitation)

Causes
- Rheumatic fever
- Congenital heart disease
- Syphilis
- Endocarditis
- Hypertension

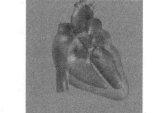

Handwritten notes:

Pericarditis: Inspiratory pain. Treat w/ NSAIDS
· Monitor for tamponade

Valvular Heart Disease

Mitral Valve Stenosis
- Early period: may have no symptoms
- Later: excessive fatigue, dyspnea on exertion, orthopnea, dry cough, hemoptysis, or pulmonary edema
- Rumbling apical diastolic murmur and a-fib are common.

Nursing and Collaborative Management
- HF care
- Monitor for a-fib with thrombus formation
- Prophylactic antibiotic therapy before any invasive procedures (dental, surgical, childbirth)
- May require surgical repair or valve replacement
- Teach that there may not be a need for lifelong anticoagulant therapy if valve replacement done

Question

The nurse has just received report on four clients. Which client should the nurse assess first?

A. A client with pericarditis with pain relieved by leaning forward
B. A client with fractured ribs with pain reported at 6/10 on a 1 to 10 scale
C. A client with stable angina who is awaiting discharge instructions
D. A client with heart failure who needs transporting for an echocardiogram

Vascular Disorders

Arterial
- Smooth, shiny skin
- Pallor on elevation
- Weak peripheral pulses
- Sharp or tingling pain
- Cool to touch
- Intermittent claudication
- Painful, nonedematous ulcers
- Bruits

Venous
- Monitor for history of deep vein thrombosis.
- Bluish-purple skin discoloration
- Normal peripheral pulses
- Warm to touch
- Slightly painful ulcers with marked edema
- Capillary refill <3 seconds
- Pruritus

Vascular Disorders: Nursing and Collaborative Management

General
- Encourage smoking cessation.
- Encourage regular exercise.
- Achieve or maintain ideal body weight.
- Follow DASH diet.
- Tight glycemic control in diabetes
- Tight BP control
- Treatment of hyperlipidemia and hypertriglyceridemia
- ACE or ARB

Arterial
- Bed rest
- Keep extremity below level of the heart.
- Topical antibiotics
- Antiplatelet agent (clopidogrel)
- Surgical grafting intervention

Venous
- Wound care
- Diet that promotes wound healing; zinc and vitamins A and C
- Compression stockings day and evening
- Teach client to elevate legs (at least 20 minutes, 4–5 times daily).

Abdominal Aortic Aneurysm

- Pulsating abdominal mass
- Bruit heard over abdomen
- Hypotension, JVD, widening pulse pressure
- Confirmed on x-ray
- If ruptures: S/S of hypovolemic shock
- Postoperative care:
  - ✓ Monitor for S/S of renal failure, MI, ARDS, or postoperative ileus
  - ✓ Changes in pulses, S/S of occluded graft (changes in pulse, pain, cyanotic extremities)

Venous Thromboembolism (VTE)

Inflammation of the venous wall with clot formation
- S/S: calf pain, induration (hardening) along the blood vessel, warmth, and redness
- Restrict ambulation
- Elevate extremity
- Antiembolic stockings
- Refrain from massaging leg muscles

Medications
- Heparin therapy: Monitor partial thromboplastin time (PTT); antidote is protamine sulfate
- Coumadin therapy: Monitor prothrombin time (PT), international normalized ratio (INR); antidote is vitamin K
- Antiplatelet agents
- Ticlopidine
- Clopidogrel bisulfate (Plavix)

* Perfusion

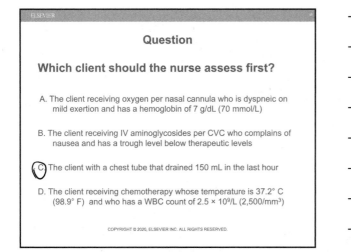

Question

Which client should the nurse assess first?

A. The client receiving oxygen per nasal cannula who is dyspneic on mild exertion and has a hemoglobin of 7 g/dL (70 mmol/L)

B. The client receiving IV aminoglycosides per CVC who complains of nausea and has a trough level below therapeutic levels

C. The client with a chest tube that drained 150 mL in the last hour

D. The client receiving chemotherapy whose temperature is 37.2° C (98.9° F) and who has a WBC count of 2.5 × 10^9/L (2,500/mm^3)

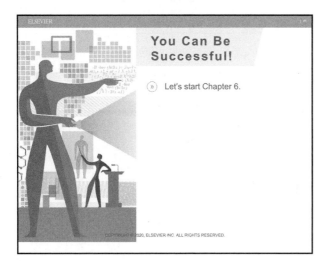

You Can Be Successful!

» Let's start Chapter 6.

Gastroesophageal Reflux Disease (GERD)

- A backward flow of stomach acid up into the esophagus
- Most common upper GI problem seen in adults and can occur in all age groups

Causes

- Predisposing conditions include:
  - Incompetent lower esophageal sphincter (LES)
  - Hiatal hernia
  - Decreased esophageal clearance (ability to clear liquids or food from the esophagus into the stomach) resulting from impaired esophageal motility
  - Decreased gastric emptying

GERD

Symptoms
- Heartburn (pyrosis) after eating
- Eructation
- Fullness and discomfort after eating
- Nocturnal coughing and wheezing
- Ask client what foods seem to aggravate symptoms.
- Positive diagnosis from barium swallow or fluoroscopy (hiatal hernia)

Laboratory Testing
- Upper GI endoscopy
- Esophagram (barium swallow)
- pH monitoring
- Motility (manometry) testing

Nursing and Collaborative Management
- Lifestyle modifications
- Encourage smoking cessation.
- Weight management
- Encourage small, frequent meals.
- Sit up while eating and remain upright for 1 hour after eating.
- Stop eating 3 hours before bedtime.
- Elevate head of bed 4 to 6 inches.
- Take proton pump inhibitors to ↓ acid production and H2.
- Take sucralfate, metoclopramide.
- Procedures to strengthen LES
- Monitor for Barrett's esophagus.

GERD Medications

- Antacids
  - Neutralize/reduce stomach acidity
- H2 receptor antagonists
  - Decrease acid secretions by blocking histamine receptors
- Proton pump inhibitors (PPIs)
  - Inhibit gastrin secretion
- Mucosal healing agents
- Promotility agents

Peptic Ulcer Disease

Significant gastric ulcers are caused by *Helicobacter pylori* bacteria.

Risk factors include:	Symptoms

• Drugs: NSAIDs, corticosteroids, aspirin
• Alcohol, coffee
• Cigarette smoking
• Stress
	• Left epigastric pain, may radiate to back
	• Symptoms occur 1 to 2 hours after meals.
	• Epigastric pain relieved with food; if penetrating, then food increases discomfort
	• Laboratory testing:
	  • Barium swallow
	  • Upper endoscopy
	  • *Helicobactor pylori* testing

Peptic Ulcer Disease

Nursing and Collaborative Management
- Onset of symptoms
- What relieves symptoms
- Monitor stools for color, consistency, occult blood
- Drug therapy includes:
  - H2 blockers
  - PPI
  - Antacids
  - Antibiotic therapy for *H. pylori*

Complications
Surgery may be needed for complications such as:
- Perforation
- Hemorrhage
- Gastric outlet obstruction

Lifestyle Changes
- Small, frequent meals
- High-fat, high-protein, low-CHO diet
- Avoid liquids with meals

Peptic Ulcer Disease

Client Teaching
Avoid medications such as:
- Salicylates
- NSAIDs

Inform HCP of h/o PUD.
Symptoms of GI bleeding:
- Dark, tarry stools
- Coffee-ground emesis
- Bright red rectal bleeding

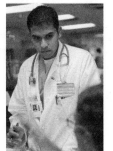

Handwritten notes:

EGD testing

If pain is UNRELIEVED by food — perforation is likely to occur.

Dumping Syndrome

Complication After Gastric Surgery

Rapid gastric emptying of hypertonic food from the stomach to the small intestine, drawing fluid into the bowel lumen, resulting in distention of the duodenum or jejunum occurs in one-third to one-half of clients following surgery.

Symptoms: nausea, vomiting, diaphoresis, explosive diarrhea, and changes in blood glucose levels

Nursing and Collaborative Management

- 6 small meals high in protein and fat and low in carbohydrates
- Eat slowly; avoid fluids during meals.
- Anticholinergic agents decrease stomach motility.
- Recline for 1 hour after eating.
- Symptoms disappear a year postop.

Question

While the nurse is obtaining the health history of a client and reviewing the medical records, which data should alert the nurse that the client has an increased risk of developing peptic ulcer disease? (Select all that apply.)

A. Excess of gastric acid or a decrease in the natural ability of the GI mucosa to protect itself from acid and pepsin

B. Invasion of the stomach and/or duodenum by *H. pylori*

C. Viral infection, allergies to certain foods, immunological factors, and psychosomatic factors

D. Taking certain drugs, including corticosteroids and antiinflammatory medications

E. Having allergies to foods containing gluten in their ingredients

---

Celiac Disease

- Causes
  - Autoimmune disease characterized by damage to the small intestinal mucosa from ingesting wheat, barley, and rye.
- Risk factors: genetic predisposition, gluten ingestion, and immune-mediated response
- Symptoms: steatorrhea, abdominal distention, and malnutrition
- Possible complications: decreased bone density, dental enamel hypoplasia, iron and folate deficiency, peripheral neuropathy, vesicular skin lesions (dermatitis herpetiformis)
- Laboratory testing: serology testing and small intestine biopsy (early diagnosis and treatment is important to prevent complications)
- Nursing and collaborative management: gluten-free diet

Crohn Disease and Ulcerative Colitis

	Crohn (Regional Enteritis)	Ulcerative Colitis
Location	Affects small and large intestines, all layers of intestine, RLQ abdominal pain DX with barium enema, capsule endoscopy	Large bowel and rectum DX with sigmoidoscopy
Symptoms	Three to four stools per day	Diarrhea, abdominal pain, 10 to 20 loose stools/day, electrolyte imbalances, anemia
Treatment	Sedatives, tranquilizers, antidiarrheals, sulfasalazine, corticosteroids, immunosuppressives, antimicrobials Surgery for complications Complication: fistula	Corticosteroids, antidiarrheals, sulfasalazine, mesalamine, infliximab, or other biological treatments
Nutrition	TPN-NPO, bland diet, no milk, vitamin and mineral supplementation	Low-residue, low-fat, high-protein diet; no dairy; calorie count; I&O

Question

The nurse is teaching a client about Crohn disease. The nurse is correct in identifying which complication as being the result of cobblestone lesions of the small intestine?

(A) Malabsorption of nutrients
B. Severe diarrhea of 15 to 20 stools per day
C. A high probability of developing intestinal cancer
D. An inability of the body to absorb water

Diverticular Diseases

Symptoms
Left lower quadrant pain
S/S of intestinal obstruction
▪Abdominal distention
▪Constipation/diarrhea
▪+ Barium enema/colonoscopy

Nursing and Collaborative Management
Sufficient fiber in diet
(avoid foods containing seeds)

If inflammation present:
▪NPO
▪Then low-residue, bland diet
▪Bulk-forming laxatives
▪Avoid heavy lifting, tight clothing, and straining

Crohn: "Cobblestone"
TPN: must have central line

Ulcerative Colitis: inflammation, wall hypertrophy. ↓ H/H — anemia

Intestinal Obstruction

Mechanical Causes
- Adhesions most common
- Strangulated hernia
- Tumors

Neurogenic Causes
- Paralytic ileus
- Spinal cord lesion

Vascular Cause
- Mesenteric artery occlusion

Symptoms
- Sudden abdominal pain
- History of obstruction
- High-pitched bowel sounds with early mechanical obstruction
- Bowel sounds diminished or absent with neurogenic or late mechanical obstruction

Nursing and Collaborative Management
- NPO
- IV fluids
- Nasogastric tube to intermittent suction

Cirrhosis

Degeneration of liver tissue

Chronic progressive disease
- Early signs: RUQ pain, fatigue
- History
  - Alcohol and/or drug abuse
  - Exposure to hepatotoxins
- Jaundice
- Fruity or musty breath
- Asterixis
- Palmar erythema
- Ascites
- Weight loss

*Refer to the review book for a complete list.

Esophageal varices may rupture and cause hemorrhage.

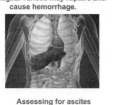

Assessing for ascites

Cirrhosis

Treatment
- Esophagogastric balloon
- Vitamin K
- Blood products
- Coagulation factors

Dietary Teaching
- Protein may have to be restricted.
- Low sodium
- Low potassium
- Low fat
- High carbohydrate
- May need to take lactulose as ammonia detoxicant/stimulant laxative

Symptoms and Nursing and Collaborative Management
- Early sign: pain RUQ quadrant
- Jaundice: yellow sclera
- Dark-colored urine; clay-colored stools
- Fruity or musty breath
- Hemodynamic stability: manage hemorrhage
- Labs: bilirubin, AST, ALT, LFH
- Avoid injections.
- Maintain pressure for 5 minutes after venipunctures.
- Monitor fluid and electrolytes.
- Vitamins K, C, folic acid

Protein ↓ in diet, then ↑
Carbs in diet.
· Bleeding precautions.

Nursing and Collaborative Management

- Monitor bleeding, avoid injections, maintain pressure 5 minutes after venipuncture, use electric razor
- Hemodynamic stability: manage hemorrhage with FFP and packed RBCs, vitamin K, H2 receptor blockers (e.g., cimetidine), and electrolyte replacements
- IV vasopressin: stops hemorrhage
  - Diuretics
  - Vitamins: K, C, folic acid
  - Lactulose as ammonia detoxicant
- Monitor fluid and electrolytes
- Maintain well-balanced, moderate-protein, high-carbohydrate diet with adequate vitamins
- Limit protein if client diagnosed with hepatic encephalopathy

Question

A client with advanced cirrhosis of the liver has an acute exacerbation of hepatic encephalopathy. Which type of food should the nurse teach the client to limit?

A. Fruits
B. Vegetables
C. Meats
D. Bread

Esophageal Varices

Causes
- Complication of cirrhosis associated with portal hypertension
- Propranolol used as preventative against rupture.
- **Rupture is a medical emergency!**

Symptoms
- Bloody vomit, stools
- Light-headedness
- Loss of consciousness
- Jaundice
- Easy bleeding, bruising
- Ascites

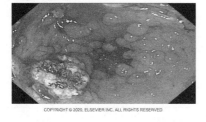

IV vasopressin COULD be use:
high risk w/ CV disorders
beta-blockers ↓ risk of
rupture

Hepatitis

Widespread inflammation of liver cells, usually caused by a virus

Viral Hepatitis

Hepatitis A

Most common, transmitted through fecal contamination, vaccine

Hepatitis B

Long-term incubation, transmitted by contaminated blood, perinatal, sexual contact, vaccine

Hepatitis C

Contaminated blood, sexual contact

Hepatitis D

Hepatitis with a coinfection with hepatitis B

Hepatitis E

Transmitted through fecal contamination, rare in United States.

Hepatitis G

Found in blood donors and can be transmitted by transfusion

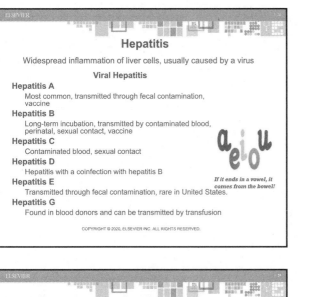

If it ends in a vowel, it comes from the bowel!

Hepatitis

Hepatitis viruses are the most common cause of hepatitis in the world, but other infections, toxic substances (e.g., alcohol, certain drugs), and autoimmune diseases may also cause hepatitis

Symptoms

Fatigue, weakness, anorexia, nausea, jaundice, dark urine, joint pain, muscle aches

Risk Groups

- Homosexual males
- IV drug users (needles)
- Tattoo/body piercing with contaminated needles
- Living in crowded conditions
- Healthcare workers employed in high-risk areas

DX: ↑ Direct bilirubin, GGT, AST, ALT, LDH, and alkaline phosphatase levels; leukopenia; hypoglycemia

Nursing and Collaborative Management

- Frequent rest periods
- Provide high-calorie, high-carbohydrate diet with moderate fats and proteins
- Administer antiemetic as needed
- Avoid alcohol intake and drugs detoxified by the liver

Pancreatitis

Acute: autodigestion of the pancreas; alcohol ingestion and biliary tract disease are major causes

Chronic: progressive, destructive disease; long-term alcohol use is major factor in disease

Symptoms

Abdominal pain is the predominant symptom of acute pancreatitis.

- Located in the LUQ
- Radiates to the back
- Sudden onset
- Described as severe, deep, piercing, and continuous
- Aggravated by eating and is not relieved by vomiting
- Accompanied by flushing, cyanosis, and dyspnea

↑ Risk of instability: fluid shift, hemorrhage in pancreas

Acute Pancreatitis

Symptoms

- Nausea and vomiting
- Low-grade fever
- Leukocytosis
- Jaundice
- Abdominal tenderness with muscle guarding
- Areas of ecchymoses, Grey Turner's spots or sign, a bluish flank discoloration, and Cullen's sign, a bluish periumbilical discoloration

- Hypotension
- Tachycardia
- Hypovolemia (massive fluid shift into the retroperitoneal space)
- Shock (hemorrhage into the pancreas)
- Toxemia (activated pancreatic enzymes)
- The lungs are frequently involved (crackles).
- Bowel sounds may be decreased or absent, and ileus may occur.

Acute Pancreatitis

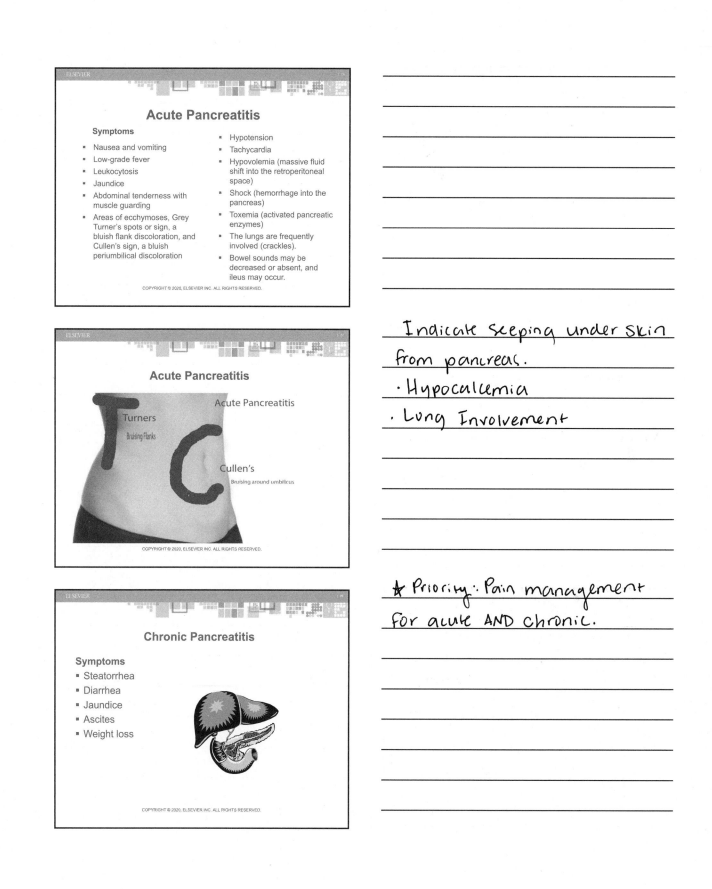

Turners — Bruising Flanks

Acute Pancreatitis

Cullen's — Bruising around umbilicus

Chronic Pancreatitis

Symptoms

- Steatorrhea
- Diarrhea
- Jaundice
- Ascites
- Weight loss

Handwritten notes:

Indicate seeping under skin from pancreas.
- Hypocalcemia
- Lung Involvement

★ Priority: Pain management for acute AND chronic.

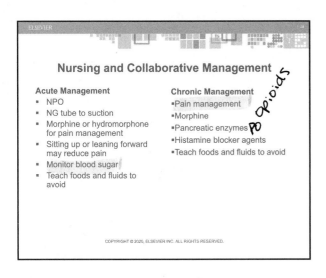

Nursing and Collaborative Management

Acute Management
- NPO
- NG tube to suction
- Morphine or hydromorphone for pain management
- Sitting up or leaning forward may reduce pain
- Monitor blood sugar
- Teach foods and fluids to avoid

Chronic Management
- Pain management *[opioids]*
- Morphine
- Pancreatic enzymes *PO*
- Histamine blocker agents
- Teach foods and fluids to avoid

Question

A client is receiving pancreatic enzyme replacement therapy for chronic pancreatitis. Which statement by the client indicates a need for more effective teaching?

- A. "I will need to mix the enzyme with a protein food." *(circled)*
- B. "I will take the enzymes with each meal."
- C. "My stools will decrease in number and frequency."
- D. "My abdominal pain may lessen."

Cholecystitis and Cholelithiasis

Cholecystitis: acute inflammation of the gallbladder
Cholelithiasis: formation or presence of gallstones

Symptoms
- Pain
- Fever
- Elevated WBCs
- Abdominal tenderness
- Jaundice

Nursing and Collaborative Management
- Analgesics for pain
- NPO
- NG to suction
- IV antibiotics
- Low-fat diet

Nursing and Collaborative Management

Cholelithiasis
- Nonsurgical removal
  - Endoscopic retrograde cholangiopancreatography (ERCP)
  - Lithotripsy
- Surgical approach
  - Cholecystectomy, laparoscopic, or open

Question

A client who is diagnosed with an obstruction of the common bile duct caused by cholelithiasis passes clay-colored stools containing streaks of fat. Which action should the nurse take?

A. Auscultate for diminished bowel sounds
B. Send a stool specimen to the lab
C. Document the assessment in the chart
D. Notify the healthcare provider

Urinary Tract Infections

- **Causes:** *Escherichia coli*, sexual intercourse, urethritis
- **Symptoms:** urinary urgency, burning sensation when urinating, cloudy urine, hematuria, pelvic pain, urine with strong odor
- Obtain clean-catch midstream specimen.
- Administer antibiotics as ordered.
- ✓ Take fully prescribed dose.
- ✓ Do not skip doses.
- Encourage fluid intake of 3000 mL/day.
- Encourage voiding every 2 to 3 hours.
- Avoid tight clothing and bubble baths.

↓ inflammation before removal of stones.
- ERCP increases risk of pancreatitis.

Urinary Tract Obstruction

Caused by calculi or stones
- Location of pain can help locate stone.
  - ✓ Flank pain (stone usually in upper ureter)
  - ✓ Pain radiating to abdomen (stone likely in ureter or bladder)

Nursing and Collaborative Management
- Administer narcotics
- Strain all urine
- Encourage high fluid intake
  - 3 to 4 L/day
- Strict I&O
- May need surgical management

Benign Prostatic Hyperplasia
Enlargement of the Prostate

Symptoms
- Increased urinary frequency
- Decreased urinary output
- Bladder distention

Nonsurgical Options for Treatment
- Can be done with laser to burn out prostate
- If prostate is too large, will use suprapubic approach
- Assess for:
  - Increased urinary frequency/decreased output
  - Bladder distention (increases risk of spasm)

Surgical Options
- Transurethral needle ablation
- Most common treatment: transurethral resection of the prostate (TURP)
- If prostate is too large, will use suprapubic approach
- Assess for:
  - Increased urinary frequency/decreased output
  - Bladder distention (increases risk of spasm)

Nursing and Collaborative Management

- Preoperative teaching
  - Pain management
  - Oversized balloon catheter
- Bladder spasms
  - Common after surgery
  - Use antispasmodics
  - ✓ Belladonna and opium suppositories
  - ✓ Oxybutynin chloride
  - ✓ Dicyclomine hydrochloride
- Continuous bladder irrigation
- Drainage should be reddish pink for 24 hours, clearing to light pink.
- Monitor color and amount of urine output.
- Notify HCP if there is ↑ bleeding and clots.

3-way irrigation
I's + O's
4-6 wk recovery time
Bladder spasms common:
antispasmodic

Discharge Teaching

- Continue to drink 12 to 14 glasses of water per day.
- Avoid straining.
- Avoid strenuous activity, sports, lifting, and intercourse for 3 to 4 weeks.
- Report large amounts of blood or frank blood.

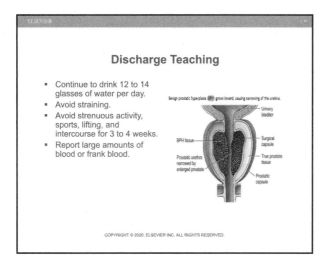

Benign prostatic hyperplasia (BPH) grows inward, causing narrowing of the urethra.
- Urinary bladder
- BPH tissue
- Surgical capsule
- Prostatic urethra narrowed by enlarged prostate
- True prostate tissue
- Prostatic capsule

Question

The charge nurse is making assignments on the renal unit. Which client should the registered nurse assign to a practical nurse who is new to the unit?

A. An older client who has thick, dark red drainage in a urinary catheter 1 day after a transurethral prostatic resection

B. A middle-aged client admitted with a diagnosis of acute renal failure secondary to a reaction to IV pyelogram dye

C. An older client who has end-stage renal disease and complains of nausea after receiving digoxin

D. A middle-aged client who receives hemodialysis and has been prescribed epoetin alfa subcutaneous daily

Question

A client is in the oliguric phase of acute kidney injury. Which findings should the nurse expect to assess in the client? (Select all that apply.)

A. 450 mL urine output in 24 hours
B. Potassium of 6.2 mEq/L
C. Sodium (serum) 155 mEq/L
D. Metabolic alkalosis
E. Weight gain

Handwritten notes:

Oliguria <400mL ⎤ 24 hr
Anuria <100 mL ⎦

In AKI: Na⁺ will drop or stay the same.
Metabolic acidosis is common

Acute Kidney Injury

A reversible syndrome if symptoms are caught early.

Remember:
- Kidneys use 25% of normal cardiac output to maintain function.
- Kidneys excrete 1 to 2 L of urine per 24 hours for adults.

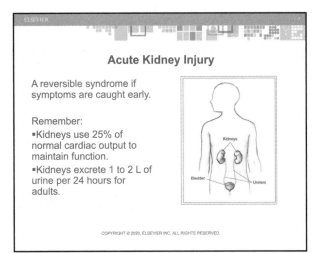

Acute Kidney Injury

Prerenal Failure
- Hemorrhage/hypovolemia
- ↓ Cardiac output
- ↓ Renal perfusion

Intrarenal Failure
- May develop secondary to prerenal failure
- Nephrotoxins, infections
- Renal injury
- Vascular lesions

Postrenal Failure
- Obstruction, calculi, BPH
- Tumors, strictures

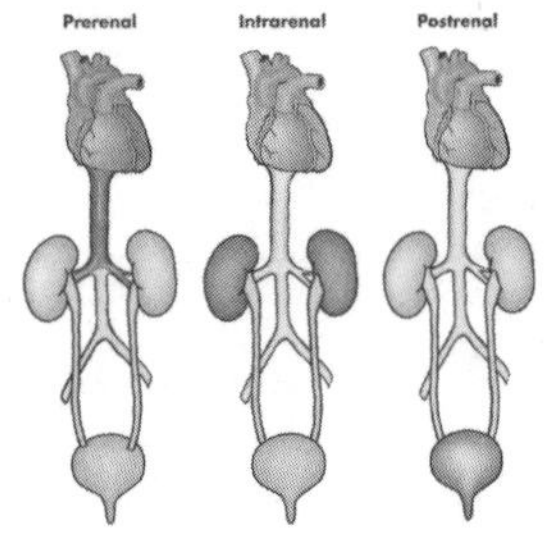

Prerenal   Intrarenal   Postrenal

Symptoms and Laboratory Testing

- ↓ Urine output
- Weight gain
- Edema
- **Diagnostic test results: Oliguric phase**
  - ↓ Urine output
  - ↑ BUN (blood urea nitrogen) and creatinine
  - ↑ Potassium
  - ↓ Sodium (serum)
  - ↓ pH
- Metabolic acidosis
- ↑ Urine sodium
- Fixed at 1.010 specific gravity

- **Diagnostic test results: Diuretic phase**
  - ↑ Urine output   4-5,000 mL
  - ↓ Fluid volume
  - ↓ Potassium
  - ↓ Sodium
  - ↓ Urine specific gravity
  - ↓ Urine sodium

- **Recovery phase:** GFR slowly increases; full recovery may take a year.

Handwritten notes:

Oliguric: 2 wk phase
Diuresis: 1 wk
Recovery: 1-1½ yrs
Strict I's + O's. q2 hr

Nursing and Collaborative Management

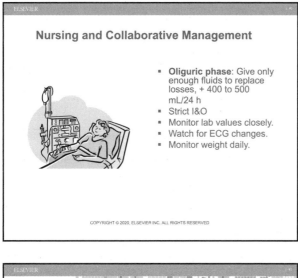

- **Oliguric phase**: Give only enough fluids to replace losses, + 400 to 500 mL/24 h
- Strict I&O
- Monitor lab values closely.
- Watch for ECG changes.
- Monitor weight daily.

Chronic Kidney Disease (CKD)

End-stage renal disease
Progressive irreversible damage to the nephrons and glomeruli

Causes
- Diabetic nephropathy
- Hypertensive nephrosclerosis
- Glomerulonephritis
- Polycystic kidney disease

Symptoms

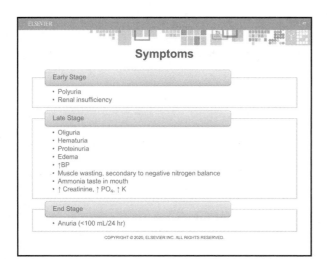

Early Stage
- Polyuria
- Renal insufficiency

Late Stage
- Oliguria
- Hematuria
- Proteinuria
- Edema
- ↑BP
- Muscle wasting, secondary to negative nitrogen balance
- Ammonia taste in mouth
- ↑ Creatinine, ↑ PO_4, ↑ K

End Stage
- Anuria (<100 mL/24 hr)

Nursing and Collaborative Management

- Monitor serum electrolytes
- Weigh daily
- Strict I&O
- Renal diet
  - Low protein
  - Low sodium
  - Low potassium
  - Low phosphate

Medications

Drugs are used to manage the associated complications.
- Aluminum hydroxide to bind phosphates
- Epoetin to treat anemia
- Antihypertensive therapy
- Calcium supplements and vitamin D
- Antihyperlipidemics
- Statins to lower LDL
- Fibrates to lower triglycerides

CAUTION: As kidney function decreases, medication doses require adjustment.

Renal Dialysis

Renal Dialysis
- Hemodialysis
  - AV fistula
- Ø Venipunctures, Ø IVs, Ø BP in AV shunt arm
- Withhold medications that would affect hemodynamic stability before dialysis

Peritoneal dialysis
- Monitor indwell and outflow times closely
- Monitor I&O

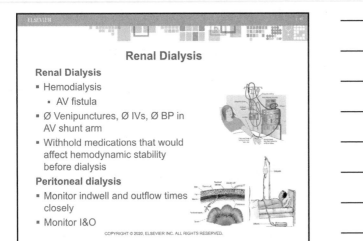

Postoperative Care: Kidney Surgery

- Auscultate to detect "wet" sounds
- Demonstrate splinting method
- Monitor for shock
- Monitor surgical site for bleeding
- Administer narcotic analgesics as needed
- Check urinary output and drainage from all tubes
- Strict I&O

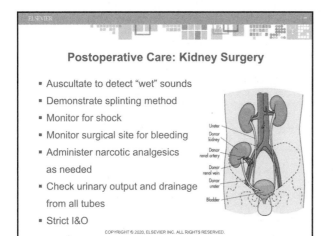

Question

After hemodialysis, the nurse is evaluating the blood results for a client who has end-stage renal disease. Which value should the nurse verify with the laboratory?

A. Elevated serum potassium
B. Increase in serum calcium
C. Low hemoglobin
D. Reduction in serum sodium

Question

A client with a 20-year history of type 1 diabetes mellitus is having renal function tests because of recent fatigue, weakness, BUN of 8.5 mmol/L (24 mg/dL), and a serum creatine of 146 mmol/L (1.6 mg/dL). Which additional early symptom of renal insufficiency should the nurse expect?

A. Dyspnea
B. Nocturia
C. Confusion
D. Stomatitis

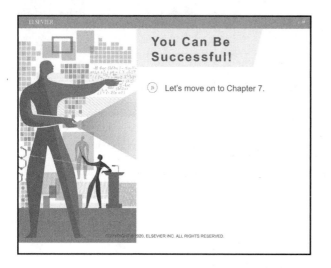

You Can Be Successful!

» Let's move on to Chapter 7.

Regulatory, Reproductive, and Urinary

Obesity, Metabolic Syndrome, Prediabetes, and Diabetes
Primary Obesity

Calorie intake exceeds the body's metabolic needs.

Abdominal and visceral fat have been linked to metabolic syndrome. Disproportionally represented in minority populations.

Assessed using BMI
- BMI of 18.5 to 24.9 kg/m²: Normal weight
- BMI of 25 to 29.9 kg/m²: Overweight
- BMI ≥30 kg/m²: Obese
- BMI >40 kg/m²: Morbidly obese

Nursing Assessment
- Risk factor screening
- Cardiovascular disease
- Hypertension
- Sleep apnea
- Type 2 diabetes

Obesity, Metabolic Syndrome, Prediabetes, and Diabetes

Lifestyle Management
- Medical/nutritional therapy
- Physical activity
- Behavior modification

Pharmacological Therapy
- Orlistat blocks fat breakdown in GI track

Metabolic Syndrome

Risk factors that ↑ an individual's chance of developing cardiovascular disease and diabetes mellitus.

Bariatric Surgery

Criteria for bariatric surgery:
- BMI ≥40 or ≥35 kg/m² with 1+ severe, obesity-related complications
- Gastric bypass, gastric banding, Roux-en-Y

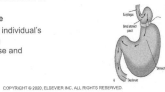

Obesity, Metabolic Syndrome, Prediabetes, and Diabetes

Nursing Assessment
Meets three or more criteria:

- ✓ **Waist circumference** ≥40 inches (102 cm) in men or ≥35 inches (88 cm) in women
- ✓ **Triglycerides** >1.7 mmol/L (>150 mg/dL) or drug treatment for elevated triglycerides
- ✓ **High-density lipoprotein (HDL) cholesterol** <0.9 mmol/L (<40 mg/dL) in men or 1.1 mmol/L (<50 mg/dL) in women or drug treatment for ↓HDL
- ✓ **BP** ≥130 mm Hg systolic or ≥85 mm Hg diastolic or drug treatment for hypertension
- ✓ **Fasting blood glucose level** ≥10 mmol/L (100 mg/dL) or drug treatment for elevated glucose

Nursing and Collaborative Management

Lifestyle management
- ✓ Medical nutritional therapy
- ✓ Physical activity
- ✓ Behavior modification

Obesity, Metabolic Syndrome, Prediabetes, and Diabetes

Prediabetes

↑ Risk for developing diabetes

Assessment

- Fasting blood glucose level of 6.1 to 6.9 mmol/L (100 to 125 mg/dL)
- 2-hour oral glucose tolerance test (OGTT) values of 7.1 to 11 mmol/L (140 to 199 mg/dL)
- Hemoglobin A_{1C}
  - Canada: 6.0% to 6.4%
  - US: 5.7% to 6.4%

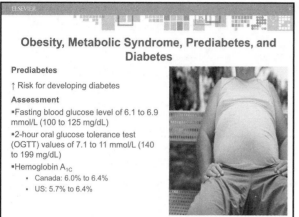

Diabetes Mellitus

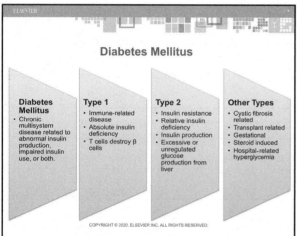

Diabetes Mellitus	Type 1	Type 2	Other Types
• Chronic multisystem disease related to abnormal insulin production, impaired insulin use, or both.	• Immune-related disease • Absolute insulin deficiency • T cells destroy β cells	• Insulin resistance • Relative insulin deficiency • Insulin production • Excessive or unregulated glucose production from liver	• Cystic fibrosis related • Transplant related • Gestational • Steroid induced • Hospital-related hyperglycemia

Diabetes: Diagnosis

A1c%	Fasting Plasma Glucose	Oral Glucose Tolerance Test
≥6.5%	≥7.0 mmol/L (≥126 mg/dL)	≥11.1 mmol/L (≥200 mg/dL)

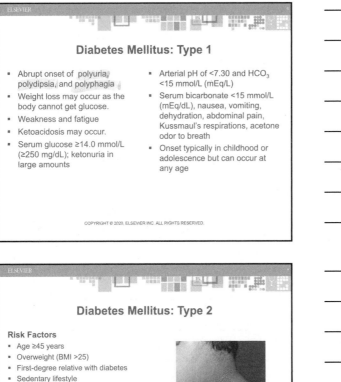

Diabetes Mellitus: Type 1

- Abrupt onset of polyuria, polydipsia, and polyphagia
- Weight loss may occur as the body cannot get glucose.
- Weakness and fatigue
- Ketoacidosis may occur.
- Serum glucose ≥14.0 mmol/L (≥250 mg/dL); ketonuria in large amounts

- Arterial pH of <7.30 and HCO₃ <15 mmol/L (mEq/L)
- Serum bicarbonate <15 mmol/L (mEq/dL), nausea, vomiting, dehydration, abdominal pain, Kussmaul's respirations, acetone odor to breath
- Onset typically in childhood or adolescence but can occur at any age

Diabetes Mellitus: Type 2

Risk Factors
- Age ≥45 years
- Overweight (BMI >25)
- First-degree relative with diabetes
- Sedentary lifestyle
- Ethnic at-risk group
- Gestational diabetes or a baby >9 lb
- CVD and/or hypertension
- Abnormal lipids (low HDL, high TG)
- Prediabetes
- PCOS
- Signs of insulin resistance (acanthosis nigricans)
- History of CV disease

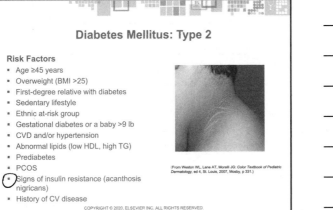

(From Weston WL, Lane AT, Morelli JG: *Color Textbook of Pediatric Dermatology*, ed 4, St. Louis, 2007, Mosby, p 331.)

Diabetes Mellitus: Type 2

- Insidious onset with the following:
- 3 Ps + fatigue + weight loss
- Recurrent infections
- Prolonged wound healing
- Visual changes
- Impotence
- Rare: ketoacidosis; more likely HHNKS with BS >33.3 mmol/L (600 mg/dL)
- Dehydration, plasma hyperosmolality, altered mental state, and absent ketone bodies

Bring glucose down slowly to minimize risk of cerebral edema.

Diabetes Mellitus: Complications

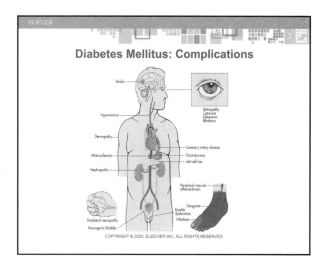

Nursing and Collaborative Management

Medical Nutrition Therapy
- Type 1: Integrate insulin with eating and exercise.
- Type 2: Heart-healthy diet and moderate weight loss of 10% to 20%
  - Space meals

Monitoring
- Detects extremes and targets
- Educate client in techniques, calibration, and record keeping.

Regular Activity
- Moderate-intensity aerobic physical activity 150 minutes/week; resistance training 3 days/week

Nursing and Collaborative Management

Education
- Injection techniques if injectable prescribed
- Refrigerate unopened insulin.
- Monitor for S/S of hypoglycemia/hyperglycemia.
- Foot care
- Manage sick days.
  - Keep taking insulin.
  - Check blood sugar more frequently.
  - Watch for S/S of hyperglycemia.

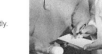

Question

The registered nurse (RN) assigns the practical nurse (PN) a client diagnosed with diabetes. Which findings should the RN instruct the PN to report immediately? (Select all that apply.)

A. Fingerstick blood sugar of 13.59 mmol/L (247 mg/dL)
B. Cold, clammy skin
C. Crackles at the end of inspiration
D. Numbness in the fingertips and toes
E. Unsteady gait, slurred speech

Diabetes Mellitus: Pharmacological Interventions

- **Sulfonylureas:** increase insulin production from the pancreas
- **Meglitinides:** increase insulin production from the pancreas
- **Biguanides:** reduce glucose production by the liver — *Metformin, glucophage*
- **a-Glucosidase inhibitors:** reduce absorption of carbohydrates
- **Thiazolidinediones:** insulin sensitizers
- **Dipeptidyl peptidase-4 inhibitor:** slows the inactivation of incretin hormones
- **Incretin mimetic:** simulates one of the incretin hormones
- **Amylin analog:** a synthetic analog of human amylin

Insulin Pharmacokinetics

Insulin	Instructions	Onset	Peak	Duration
Glulisine (Apidra)	Given within 15 minutes of meal	0.25 h	1 h	2 to 3 h
Lispro (Humalog)	Given within 15 minutes of meal	0.25 h	1 h	4 h
Aspart (NovoLog)	Given within 15 minutes of meal	0.5 h	1 to 3 h	3 to 5 h
Regular (Humulin R)	Given within 30 minutes of meal	0.5 to 1 h	2 to 4 h	5 to 7 h
NPH (Humulin N)	Can be mixed with rapid-acting insulins	1 to 2 h	4 to 12 h	16 to 24 h
Glargine (Lantus)	Usually given once a day in the morning	1 to 5 h	Plateau	24 h
Detemir (Levemir)	Acts as basal insulin	3 to 4 h	Peakless	24 h

→ IV (Regular Humulin R)
→ Cloudy (NPH Humulin N)

- Afrezza: inhaled insulin
  Fast-acting

Long-Acting Insulin

- Cannot be mixed with any other type of insulin
  - Usually given once daily in the morning
  - Administer 4 hours either before or after contrast x-ray.
  - Do NOT shake solutions.
  - CAUTION: Clear colored; do not confuse with regular insulin
- Glargine (Lantus)
  - Onset 1 to 5 hours; peak: plateau; duration 24 hours
- Detemir (Levemir):
  - Onset 3 to 4 hours; peakless; duration 24 hours

Question

The nurse is reviewing the current medication list of a client, newly diagnosed with type 1 diabetes, who will be prescribed insulin. Which medications should the RN discuss with the healthcare provider? (Select all that apply.)

A. Prednisone
B. Atenolol
C. Clarithromycin
D. Acetaminophen
E. Ibuprofen
F. Pantoprazole sodium

Question

A client who was recently prescribed metformin hydrochloride calls the clinic to discuss symptoms of bloating, nausea, cramping, and diarrhea. Which instructions should the nurse provide the client? (Select all that apply.)

A. Discontinue the medication immediately
B. Increase fiber and fluids in the diet
C. Monitor the symptoms
D. Continue to take the metformin as prescribed
E. Seek immediate emergency medical care

T3 > 220   T4 > 12

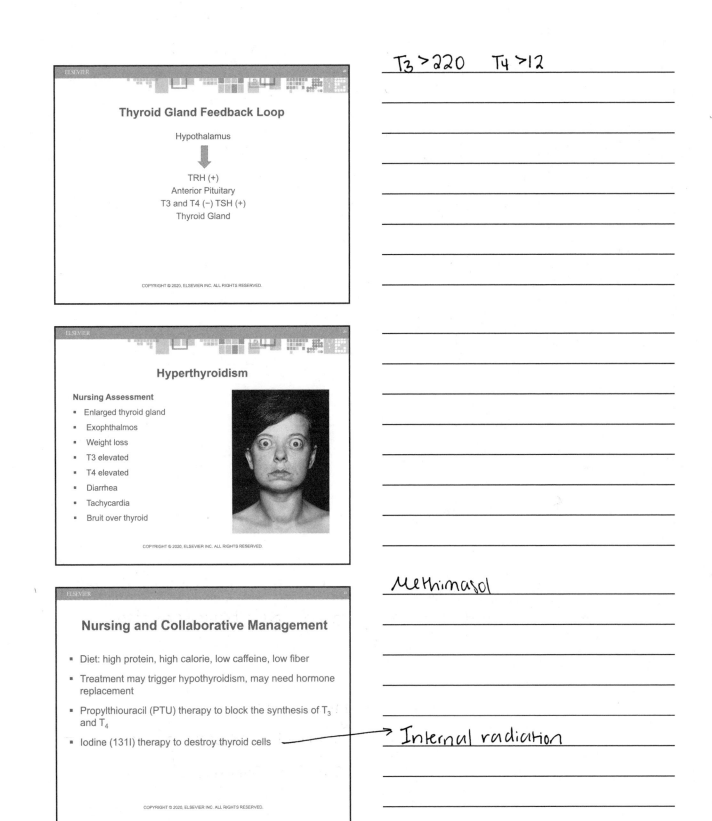

Thyroid Gland Feedback Loop

Hypothalamus

⬇

TRH (+)
Anterior Pituitary
T3 and T4 (−) TSH (+)
Thyroid Gland

Hyperthyroidism

Nursing Assessment

- Enlarged thyroid gland
- Exophthalmos
- Weight loss
- T3 elevated
- T4 elevated
- Diarrhea
- Tachycardia
- Bruit over thyroid

Nursing and Collaborative Management

- Diet: high protein, high calorie, low caffeine, low fiber
- Treatment may trigger hypothyroidism, may need hormone replacement
- Propylthiouracil (PTU) therapy to block the synthesis of T_3 and T_4
- Iodine (131I) therapy to destroy thyroid cells

Methimazol

→ Internal radiation

Hyperthyroidism: Surgical Management

Thyroidectomy

- Position in high Fowler's
- Check behind neck for drainage
- Support neck when moving client
- Assess for laryngeal edema
- Have tracheotomy set, oxygen, and suction equipment at bedside
- Have calcium gluconate at bedside

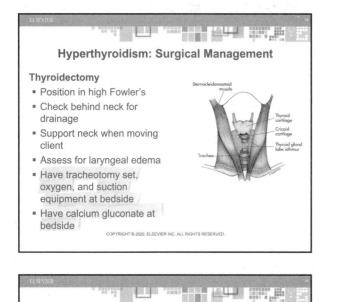

Sternocleidomastoid muscle
Thyroid cartilage
Cricoid cartilage
Thyroid gland lobe isthmus
Trachea

Hypothyroidism

Nursing Assessment

- Fatigue
- Bradycardia
- Weight gain
- Constipation
- Periorbital edema
- Cold intolerance ✗
- Low T_3 (<70 ng/dL)
- Low T_4 (<5 ng/dL)

Hypothyroidism

Medications
- Levothyroxine (Synthroid)
- ✓ Monitor heart rate
- ✓ Hold for pulse >100 beats/min
- Liothyronine (Cytomel)
- ✓ Increase metabolic rate
- ✓ Act as synthetic T3
- ✓ Check hormone levels regularly
- ✓ Avoid food containing iodine
- Levothyroxine (T4) + liothyronine (T3) (Liotrix)
- ✓ Fast onset

Nursing and Collaborative Treatment
- Myxedema coma: an acute exacerbation of hypothyroidism; maintain airway
- Teach medication regimen
- Monitor for side effects of medications
- Monitor bowel program for signs/symptoms of constipation

Levothyroxine: Take 1st thing a.m. SE: tachycardia

{ fast-acting
Liotrix: myexedema coma — airway concern

Question

Which client should the nurse assess first?

A. The client diagnosed with hyperthyroidism who is exhibiting exophthalmos

B. The client diagnosed with type 1 diabetes who has an inflamed foot ulcer

C. The client with Cushing syndrome exhibiting moon face

D. The client with Addison disease showing tremors and diaphoresis

→ Indicates drop in glucose — emergent!

Question

Which adaptation of the environment is most important for the nurse to include in the plan of care for a client diagnosed with myxedema?

A. Reduce environmental stimuli
B. Prevent direct sunlight from entering the room
C. Maintain a warm room temperature
D. Minimize exposure to visitors

Question

The nurse suspects a postoperative thyroidectomy client may have had an inadvertent removal of the parathyroid when the client begins to experience which symptoms? (Select all that apply.)

A. Hematoma formation

B. Harsh, vibratory sounds on inspiration

C. Tingling of lips, hands, and toes

D. Positive Chvostek's sign

E. Sensation of fullness at the incision site

Addison Disease

Etiology
- Sudden withdrawal from corticosteroids
- Hypofunction of adrenal cortex
- Lack of pituitary ACTH

Signs and Symptoms
- Weight loss, N/V
- Hypovolemia, hypoglycemia
- Hyponatremia, hyperkalemia
- Loss of body hair
- Postural hypotension
- Hyperpigmentation

Collaborative Management
- Frequent vital signs
- Weigh daily
- Monitor serum electrolytes
- Diet: high sodium, low potassium, high carbohydrates
- At least 3 L of fluid per day
- Wear medic alert bracelet
- Monitor for symptoms of overdosage/underdosage of corticosteroid and mineralocorticoid therapy
- Carry emergency kit with 100 mg intramuscular corticosteroid

Question

A client is admitted with a diagnosis of Addison's crisis. The nurse places a peripheral saline lock. Which prescription(s) provided by the HCP should be questioned? (Select all that apply.)

A. IV D5NS at 300 mL/h for 3 hours
B. Hydrocortisone sodium succinate 100 mg IV push
C. Potassium 20 mEq in 100 mL saline IV over 60 minutes
D. 50% dextrose intravenous push
E. 10% calcium chloride 5 mL intravenously over 10 minutes

Cushing Syndrome: Nursing Assessment

Excess adrenal corticoid activity caused by adrenal, pituitary, or hypothalamus tumors

- Moon face
- Edema of lower extremities
- Flat affect
- Obesity
- Abdominal striae
- Buffalo hump (fat deposits)
- Muscle atrophy, weakness
- Thin, dry, pale skin
- Hypertension

- Osteoporosis
- Immunosuppressed ☆ *priority*
- Hypervolemia
- Hirsutism
- Lab results
  - Hyperglycemia
  - Hypernatremia
  - Hypokalemia
  - Increased plasma cortisol levels

Handwritten notes:

Addisonian crisis: vascular collapse. Emergent injection of corticosteroids.
- Glucose, hydration, corticosteroids.

Nursing and Collaborative Management

- Monitor for S/S of infection.
- Fever
- Skin lesions
- Elevated WBCs
- Wear medic alert bracelet.
- Avoid extreme temperatures, infections, emotional disturbances.
- Diet:

✓Low sodium; low carbohydrate

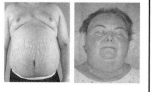

Sexually Transmitted Infections (STIs)

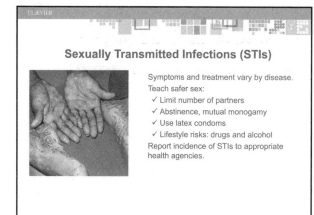

Symptoms and treatment vary by disease.
Teach safer sex:
- ✓ Limit number of partners
- ✓ Abstinence, mutual monogamy
- ✓ Use latex condoms
- ✓ Lifestyle risks: drugs and alcohol

Report incidence of STIs to appropriate health agencies.

Teaching to prevent transmission.

Sexually Transmitted Infections (STIs)

- Syphilis
- Gonorrhea
- Chlamydia
- Trichomonas
- Candidiasis
- Herpes
- Human papillomavirus
- HIV/AIDS

→ precancerous

Question

A client who had an abdominal hysterectomy for cervical adenocarcinoma in situ is preparing for discharge. Which recommendation about women's health screening examinations should the nurse offer?

A. Continue the annual Pap smear and mammogram, biannual clinical breast examinations, and monthly breast self-examinations (BSE).

B. A Pap smear is no longer necessary, but continue the annual mammogram and biannual clinical breast examinations, plus monthly BSE.

C. If the ovaries have been removed, only an annual mammogram and clinical breast examinations are necessary.

D. Annual mammograms are not needed if biannual breast examinations and weekly BSE are performed.

Benign Uterine Tumors

Fibroids

Arise from uterine muscle tissue
- Fertility issues
- Menorrhagia
- Uterine enlargement
- Dysmenorrhea
- Anemia
- Low back and pelvic pain
- Tend to disappear after menopause

Nonsurgical option: magnetic resonance-guided focused ultrasound

Surgical options: Myomectomy, hysterectomy; fertility concerns

Post-op Myomectomy / hysterectomy
Saturated pad q3 hrs —
Check BP for hypovolemia.

Question

A client with menopause reports that since stopping hormone replacement therapy (HRT), she has had increased vaginal discomfort during intercourse. Which action should the nurse take?

A. Suggest the use of vaginal cream or lubricant

B. Recommend that the client abstain from sexual intercourse

C. Teach the client to perform Kegel exercises daily

D. Instruct the client to resume HRT

Bowel | Bladder repairs

Pelvic Organ Prolapse (POP): Uterine Prolapse, Cystocele, and Rectocele

Preventive measures
- Postpartum perineal exercises (Kegel)
- Spaced pregnancy
- Weight control

Differing S/S for each condition

Surgical Intervention
- Hysterectomy
- Anterior and posterior vaginal repair

Manage postoperative pain

Monitor postoperative urinary output

Observe for S/S of bleeding and infection postoperative

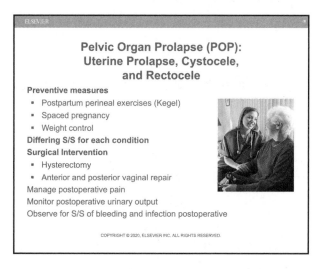

Question

A client who had a vaginal hysterectomy the previous day is saturating perineal pads with blood that require frequent changes during the night. Which priority action should the nurse take?

A. Provide iron-rich foods on each dietary tray

B. Monitor the client's vital signs every 2 hours

C. Administer IV fluids at the prescribed rate

D. Encourage postoperative leg exercises

Question

The nurse assigned to the women's health unit received the morning report. Which client should the nurse assess first?

A. A 49-year-old client 1-day postvaginal hysterectomy who is saturating pads every 3 hours

B. A 34-year-old client postuterine artery embolization who has not voided since her indwelling catheter was removed 4 hours ago

C. A 52-year-old client who is 2 days postabdominal hysterectomy requesting oral analgesics instead of the PCA pump

D. A 67-year-old client 1-day postanterior and posterior repair who is refusing to ambulate with the unlicensed assistive personnel (UAP)

Male Reproductive Conditions: Prostatitis

Prostatitis is one of the most common urologic disorders.

Common manifestations of acute bacterial prostatitis include the following:
- Fever
- Chills
- Back pain
- Perineal pain
- Dysuria
- Urinary frequency
- Urgency
- Cloudy urine

Diagnostic Studies
- Urinalysis (UA)
- Urine culture
- White blood cells (WBCs)
- Blood cultures
- PSA test (may be done to rule out prostate cancer)

Male Reproductive Conditions: Prostatitis

Nursing and Collaborative Management

Antibiotics
- Trimethoprim and sulfamethoxazole (Bactrim)
- Ciprofloxacin (Cipro)
- Ofloxacin (Floxin)
- Doxycycline (Vibramycin)
- Tetracycline

Antiinflammatory agents for pain control

Encourage fluid intake

More hydrated = more comfortable

Erectile Dysfunction

Erectile Dysfunction (ED)
The inability to attain or maintain an erect penis that allows satisfactory sexual performance.

Etiology

- Diabetes
- Vascular disease
- Side effects from medications
- Result of surgery (prostatectomy)
- Trauma

- Chronic illness
- Drugs and alcohol
- Stress/depression
- Difficulty in a relationship
- Decreased gonadal hormone secretion

Erectile Dysfunction: Oral Drug Therapy

Sildenafil citrate

Dosage: 25 to 100 mg po, one dose/day, 1 hour before sexual activity

- May potentiate the hypotensive effect of nitrates
- They are contraindicated for individuals taking nitrates (e.g., nitroglycerin) and riociguat.
- Teach clients to seek medical attention for an erection lasting longer than 4 hours (priapism).
- Use with caution in elderly because drugs are slow to metabolize and be excreted.

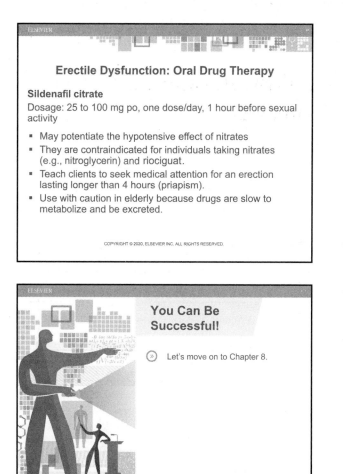

You Can Be Successful!

» Let's move on to Chapter 8.

8 Movement, Coordination, and Sensory Input

Level of Consciousness

- Glasgow Coma Scale
- ✓ Used to assess level of consciousness (LOC)
- ✓ Maximum score 15, minimum 3
- ✓ Score of ≤7 = coma
- ✓ Score of 3 to 4 = high mortality rate
- ✓ Score of >8 = good prognosis
- A decrease in LOC may be in the earliest sign of increasingly intracranial pressure (ICP).
- Neurological vital signs
- ✓ Pupil size
- ✓ Limb movement
- ✓ Vital signs

GLASGOW COMA SCALE*	
Eye Opening	
Spontaneous	4
To sound	3
To pain	2
Never	1
Motor Response	
Obeys commands	6
Localizes pain	5
Normal flexion (withdrawal)	4
Abnormal flexion	3
Extension	2
None	1
Verbal Response	
Oriented	5
Confused conversation	4
Inappropriate words	3
Incomprehensible sounds	2
None	1
* The highest possible score is 15	

Handwritten note: Pupils dilate on the side of injury.

Nursing Assessment

Assess for early signs/symptoms of changes in LOC, which is the most sensitive and reliable indicator.

Early signs
- ↓ LOC
- Change in orientation

Late signs
- Cushing's triad

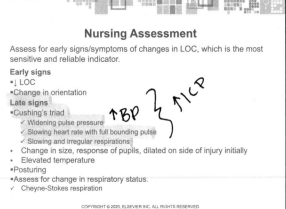

Handwritten note: ↑BP } ↑ICP

  - ✓ Widening pulse pressure
  - ✓ Slowing heart rate with full bounding pulse
  - ✓ Slowing and irregular respirations
- Change in size, response of pupils, dilated on side of injury initially
- Elevated temperature
- Posturing
- Assess for change in respiratory status.
  - ✓ Cheyne-Stokes respiration

Handwritten note: ICP: norm 5-15
★ Mannitol (diuretic) for ICP

Nursing and Collaborative Management

- Maintain airway and provide adequate oxygenation.
- ↓ LOC will need mechanical ventilation
  - ✓ Hyperventilate before suctioning.
  - ✓ Limit suctioning to 15 seconds.
  - ✓ Keep airway free of secretions.
  - ✓ Prevent aspiration; turn head to side.
  - ✓ Elevate HOB to 30 degrees to enhance respiration.

1) Dexamethasone (Decadron)
· Ø narcotics: ↓ Loc — deters early identification.

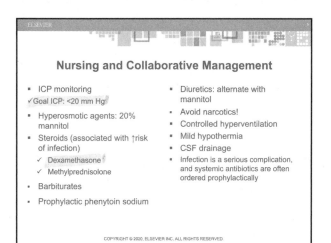

Nursing and Collaborative Management

- ICP monitoring
- ✓ Goal ICP: <20 mm Hg
- Hyperosmotic agents: 20% mannitol
- Steroids (associated with ↑risk of infection)
  - ✓ Dexamethasone
  - ✓ Methylprednisolone
- Barbiturates
- Prophylactic phenytoin sodium

- Diuretics: alternate with mannitol
- Avoid narcotics!
- Controlled hyperventilation
- Mild hypothermia
- CSF drainage
- Infection is a serious complication, and systemic antibiotics are often ordered prophylactically

Question

The nurse is caring for several clients. Which client should the nurse assess first?

A. A 20-year-old client whose Glasgow Coma Scale is 8 and unchanged from the last assessment

B. A 45-year-old client with a left-sided cerebrovascular accident (CVA) who refuses his morning care

C. A 38-year-old client who is increasingly stuporous after an aneurysm repair

D. A 29-year-old client post motor vehicle accident (MVA) whose Glasgow Coma Scale was 9 one hour ago and is now 10

Question

Which change in the status of a client being treated for increased intracranial pressure warrants immediate action by the nurse?

A. Urinary output changes from 20 to 50 mL/h

B. Arterial PCO_2 changes from 40 to 30 mm Hg

C. Glasgow Coma Scale score changes from 5 to 7

D. Pulse drops from 88 to 68 beats/min

Head Injury

Symptoms

- Changes in LOC
- Signs of increased intracranial pressure (ICP)
- ✓ Changes in VS
- ✓ Headache, amnesia
- ✓ Vomiting
- ✓ Pupillary changes (unequal/dilated)
- ✓ Seizure
- ✓ Ataxia
- ✓ Abnormal posturing (decorticate [A] or decerebrate [B])
- ✓ Extremity motor strength and use: depressed or hyperactive
- ✓ Check for lacerations, bruises, skull depression, confusion, combativeness, personality changes

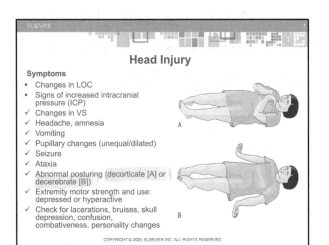

CSF Leakage

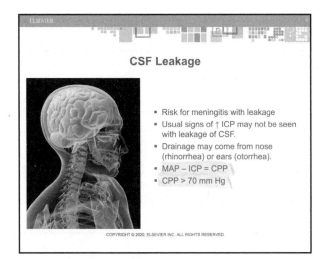

- Risk for meningitis with leakage
- Usual signs of ↑ ICP may not be seen with leakage of CSF.
- Drainage may come from nose (rhinorrhea) or ears (otorrhea).
- MAP – ICP = CPP
- CPP > 70 mm Hg

Nursing and Collaborative Management

- Neurological assessment every 15 minutes
- Notify MD at *first* sign of deterioration
- Limit visitors
- Decrease stimuli
- Prevent straining
- Keep HOB at 30 to 45 degrees
- Avoid neck flexion
- Monitor I&O

Keep legs straight

Stroke (Brain Attack) or Cerebrovascular Accident

- Hemorrhage into brain tissue
  - Ischemic stroke
  - ✓ Thromboembolic clot
  - ✓ Embolic clot

Transient ischemic attack (TIA) is a temporary episode of neurological dysfunction lasting less than 1 hour. (Most fully resolve.)

Nursing Assessment

- Risk factors
  - CVD, hypertension, previous TIA
  - Diabetes
  - Advanced age, males, African American
  - History of a-fib or flutter
  - BCPs, hormone replacement, antihistamine drugs
  - Smoking, alcohol, substance abuse
- Symptoms
  - Hemiparesis, hemiplegia
  - Dysarthria, dysphasia, aphasia, apraxia
  - Sensory disturbances
  - Impaired mental capacity/psychological loss
  - Bladder dysfunction
  - FAST

Nursing and Collaborative Management

- ✓ Time lost is brain lost.
- ✓ Hemorrhagic or ischemic
- ✓ CT scan or MRI
- ✓ Prepare for thrombolytic therapy (limited therapeutic window).
- ✓ Assess for signs and symptoms of increased ICP.
- ✓ Assess verbal ability and plan care appropriate to client's ability to communicate.
- ✓ Assess swallowing to prevent aspiration.
- ✓ Assess for bowel and bladder control.
- ✓ Assess functional abilities.
  - ✓ Mobility, ADLs, elimination

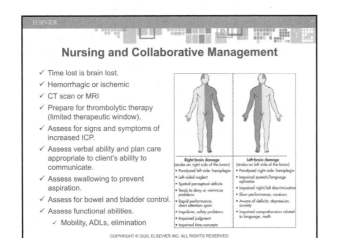

Right-brain damage (stroke on right side of the brain)	Left-brain damage (stroke on left side of the brain)
• Paralyzed left side: hemiplegia	• Paralyzed right side: hemiplegia
• Left-sided neglect	• Impaired speech/language aphasias
• Spatial-perceptual deficits	• Impaired right/left discrimination
• Tends to deny or minimize problems	• Slow performance, cautious
• Rapid performance, short attention span	• Aware of deficits: depression, anxiety
• Impulsive, safety problems	• Impaired comprehension related to language, math
• Impaired judgment	
• Impaired time concepts	

Handwritten notes:

FAST — 3hr timeframe
Face, Arms, Speech, Time

CAT/MRI scan
- Clot: thrombolytics/stent
- bleed: coils to stop bleed, craniotomy.
★ Rehabilitation: Start from head + work your way down.
Ex. airway, communication, swallow

Question

The nurse is planning a class on stroke prevention for clients with hypertension. Which information reflects accurate prevention measures that the clients can undertake? (Select all that apply.)

A. Limit salt intake to 1500 mg/day or less ⟲
B. Eliminate tobacco products ⟲
C. Initiate a program of walking 1 mile per day ⟲
D. Achieve a body mass index (BMI) of 26.2
E. Schedule routine health assessments biannually

Question

Which client should be assigned to a graduate nurse orienting to the neurological unit?

A. A client with a head injury who has a Glasgow Coma Scale of 6

B. A client who developed autonomic dysreflexia after a T6 spinal cord injury

C. A client with multiple sclerosis who needs the first dose of interferon ⟲

D. A client diagnosed with Guillain-Barré syndrome

Question

Which findings by the nurse indicate an early sign of increased ICP in a client newly diagnosed with a cerebral vascular accident? (Select all that apply.)

A. Alteration in the ability to respond to questions ⟲
B. Alteration in the ability to respond to verbal stimuli ⟲
C. Consensual response of pupils
D. Heart rate 50, blood pressure 192/60 ⟲ *late sign*
E. Drooping of the mouth on one side

Parkinson's Disease

Symptoms

Rigidity

Masklike face

Akinesia
-Difficulty initiating and continuing movement
-Bradykinesia
Tremors
-Resting
-Pill rolling
Postural instability

Nursing and Collaborative Management
- *Safety is always a priority!*
- Take medications with meals.
- Administer promptly.
- Change positions slowly to decrease postural hypotension.
- Thicken liquids.
- Provide soft, ground foods.
- Encourage activity and exercise.

Parkinson Disease: Medications

- **Dopaminergics**
  - ✓ Levodopa
  - ✓ Blocks breakdown of levodopa to allow more levodopa to cross the blood-brain barrier
  - ✓ Avoid foods high in vitamin B$_6$ and protein
  - ✓ Levodopa-carbidopa oral
  - ✓ Allows for less use of levodopa and helps decrease side effects
- **Dopaminergic Agonists**
  - • Help with motor fluctuations
  - • Rotigotine, pramipexole, ropinirole, amantadine, apomorphine

- **Anticholinergics**
  - ✓ Treat tremors
  - ✓ Trihexyphenidyl
  - ✓ Benztropine mesylate
  - ✓ Procyclidine hydrochloride
- **Antihistamine**
  - ✓ Diphenhydramine
- **Monoamine Oxidase Inhibitors**
  - ✓ Selegiline
- **Catechol-O-methyl transferase (COMT) inhibitors**
  - ✓ Entacapone

Question

The nurse is providing safety education to a client diagnosed with Parkinson disease who is prescribed carbidopa-levodopa. The nurse knows that safety education has been effective when the client verbalizes which statement? (Select all that apply.)

A. "I will take the medication at bedtime."
B. "I will apply sunscreen before I walk outdoors."
C. "It's OK for me to eat tuna on whole wheat toast and a banana."
D. "I will take the medication on an empty stomach early in the morning."
E. "I will remember to keep hydrated and monitor urine output."

Handwritten notes

Rigidity, Akinesia, Tremor
1) prevention of aspiration
2) ambulation Safety
prone to orthostatic hypotension
· Psychosocial Support: keep social.

VB6: grain foods

taken 3-4x/day
taken w/ food (not protein / B6)

Guillain-Barré Syndrome

Involves peripheral and cranial nerves in acute inflammatory demyelination process

Nursing Assessment

- Usually occurs after an upper respiratory infection
- Ascending paralysis
- Rapid demyelination of the nerves
- Paralysis of respiratory system may occur quickly.
- Prepare to intubate.
- Some clients experience a prolonged recovery time

Nursing and Collaborative Management

- ✓ Plasmapheresis over 10 to 15 days
- ✓ IV high-dose immunoglobulin (Sandoglobulin) is effective as plasma exchange and has the advantage of immediate availability and greater safety
- ✓ Maintain patent airway
- ✓ Reposition frequently
- ✓ Impaired swallowing may need TPN or NPO if gag reflex is absent
- ✓ Supervise small, frequent feedings; thicken liquids
- ✓ Provide psychological support

IGg: hydrated and good kidney function.

Question

The nurse is caring for a client with Guillain-Barré syndrome. Which information should the nurse report to the primary healthcare provider?

- A. Ascending numbness from the feet to the knees
- B. A decrease in cognitive status
- C. Blurred vision and sensation changes
- D. A persistent unilateral headache

Multiple Sclerosis

Demyelination of the central nervous system

Symptoms

- Messages garbled, short-circuited from brain to CNS
- Clients experience periods of remissions and exacerbations.
- Changes in visual field, diplopia
- Weaknesses in extremities
- Numbness, tremors
- Visual or swallowing difficulties
- Severe fatigue/emotional problems
- Gait disturbances

Nursing and Collaborative Management

- Encourage self-care, rest periods
- Initiate fall prevention
- Implement voiding schedule, bowel regimen
- Refer to home care
- Administer steroids, chemotherapeutic drugs

Age: 20-40
1) prevention aspiration
2) safe ambulation
3) Vision changes

Pharmacological Therapy

Corticosteroids
- ACTH
- Prednisone
- Methylprednisolone

Immunomodulators
- Interferon-beta
- Glatiramer acetate

Immunosuppressants
- Mitoxantrone HCL

Cholinergics
- Bethanechol
- Neostigmine

Anticholinergics
- Propantheline bromide
- Oxybutynin

Muscle Relaxants
- Diazepam
- Baclofen
- Dantrolene sodium
- Tizanidine

CNS Stimulants
- Methylphenidate HCL
- Modafinil
- Pemoline

Antiviral/Antiparkinsonian Drugs
- Amantadine

Myasthenia Gravis

- A chronic neuromuscular autoimmune disease
- Causes
- ✓ Fluctuating muscle weakness and abnormal fatigue of voluntary muscles that increase throughout the day

Symptoms
- Ocular muscle weakness
- Bulbar muscle weakness — *Weak cough / gag*
- Skeletal muscle weakness

Myasthenia Gravis

Diagnosis
- Based on clinical presentation
- Muscle weakness
- Confirmed by improved response to anticholinesterase drugs
- Tensilon test: 2 mg IV given in small doses

Nursing and Collaborative Management
- Anticholinesterase agents
  - Try to achieve maximum strength and endurance.
  - Block action of cholinesterase.
  - Increase levels of ACH at junctions.
  - Common medications: mestinon, prostigmin
  - Start with minimal doses
  - ✓ Onset 30 minutes
  - ✓ Duration 3 to 4 hours
  - ✓ Must take on time!
- Corticosteroid: prednisone
- Immunosuppressive agents: azathioprine, cyclophosphamide

Tensilon: muscle weakness should IMPROVE

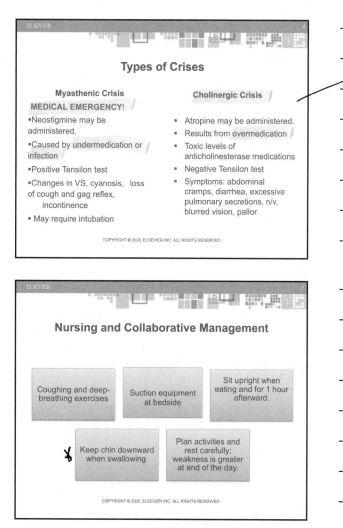

Types of Crises

Myasthenic Crisis
MEDICAL EMERGENCY!

- Neostigmine may be administered.
- Caused by undermedication or infection
- Positive Tensilon test
- Changes in VS, cyanosis, loss of cough and gag reflex, incontinence
- May require intubation

Cholinergic Crisis

- Atropine may be administered.
- Results from overmedication
- Toxic levels of anticholinesterase medications
- Negative Tensilon test
- Symptoms: abdominal cramps, diarrhea, excessive pulmonary secretions, n/v, blurred vision, pallor

→ Intervene: atropine sulfate

Nursing and Collaborative Management

Coughing and deep-breathing exercises	Suction equipment at bedside	Sit upright when eating and for 1 hour afterward.
Keep chin downward when swallowing.	Plan activities and rest carefully; weakness is greater at end of the day.	

Spinal Cord Injury

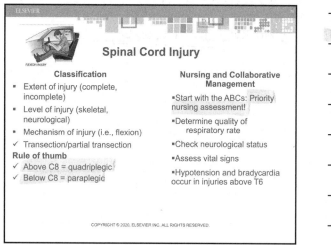

Classification

- Extent of injury (complete, incomplete)
- Level of injury (skeletal, neurological)
- Mechanism of injury (i.e., flexion)
- ✓ Transection/partial transection

Rule of thumb
- ✓ Above C8 = quadriplegic
- ✓ Below C8 = paraplegic

Nursing and Collaborative Management

- Start with the ABCs: Priority nursing assessment!
- Determine quality of respiratory rate
- Check neurological status
- Assess vital signs
- Hypotension and bradycardia occur in injuries above T6

C3-C5: airway
T5-T6: neurogenic shock —
autonomic dysreflexia
Seen: hypotension, ↓ ♡ rate

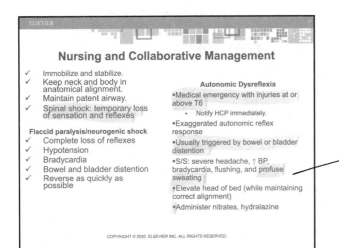

Nursing and Collaborative Management

- ✓ Immobilize and stabilize.
- ✓ Keep neck and body in anatomical alignment.
- ✓ Maintain patent airway.
- ✓ Spinal shock: temporary loss of sensation and reflexes

Flaccid paralysis/neurogenic shock
- ✓ Complete loss of reflexes
- ✓ Hypotension
- ✓ Bradycardia
- ✓ Bowel and bladder distention
- ✓ Reverse as quickly as possible

Autonomic Dysreflexia
- ▪ Medical emergency with injuries at or above T6
  - ▪ Notify HCP immediately.
- ▪ Exaggerated autonomic reflex response
- ▪ Usually triggered by bowel or bladder distention
- ▪ S/S: severe headache, ↑ BP, bradycardia, flushing, and profuse sweating
- ▪ Elevate head of bed (while maintaining correct alignment)
- ▪ Administer nitrates, hydralazine

Nursing and Collaborative Management

- ▪ Monitor for paralytic ileus.
  - ✓ Assess bowel sounds.
- ▪ Kinetic bed to promote blood flow, ROM exercises
- ▪ Anti-embolism stockings, sequential compression devices
- ▪ Protect from skin breakdown.
- ▪ Psychosocial assessment
- ▪ Bowel and bladder training
  - ▪ Keep bladder empty and urine dilute and acidic to prevent urinary tract infection

Fractures: Nursing Assessment

Symptoms and Assessment
- ▪ Swelling, deformity of the extremity
- ▪ Discoloration, loss of functional ability
- ▪ Fracture evident on x-ray
- ▪ Assess for 5 Ps of neurovascular functioning.
  - ✓ Pain, Paresthesia, Pulse, Pallor, and Paralysis
- ▪ Assess neurovascular area distal to injury.
  - ✓ Skin color, temperature, sensation, capillary refill, mobility, pain, pulses, compartment syndrome

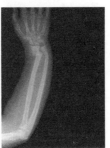

Handwritten notes:

Neurogenic shock: bradycardia
Cause: spinal cord compression—
emergent. (After 12hr → permanent)

→ Profuse sweating ① sign:
above injury. ↑ BP: risk HTN
stroke.

Stabilize → Rehabilitate

(6) Poikilothermia: inability to regulate
temp to fractured area.

36 hr window: ↑ risk for fat embolism.

Nursing and Collaborative Management

- Instruct client on proper use of assistive devices.
- Closed or open reduction
- Postreduction
  - ✓ Cast
  - ✓ Traction
  - ✓ External fixation
  - ✓ Splints
  - ✓ Orthoses (braces)

Question

The nurse is assessing a client who is scheduled for surgical fixation of a compound fracture of the right ulna. Which finding should the nurse report to the healthcare provider?

A. Ecchymosis around the fracture site
B. Crepitus at the fracture site
C. Paresthesia distal to the fracture site
D. Diminished range of motion of the right arm

Joint Replacement

- **After Surgery**
  - Check circulation, sensation, and movement of extremity distal to replacement area.
  - Keep body in proper alignment.
  - Encourage fluid intake.
  - Use of bedpan, commode chair
  - Coordinate rehabilitation process.
- **Instructions for Discharge Home**
  - Safety
  - Accessibility
- **Drugs**
  - Anticoagulants
  - Analgesics
  - Parenteral antibiotics

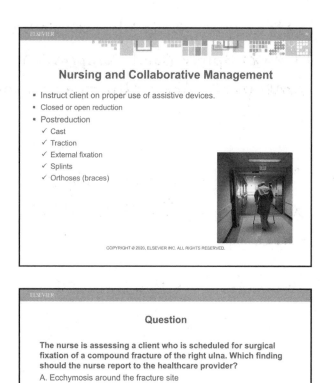

Amputation

Postoperative Care

- Monitor surgical dressing for drainage.
- Proper body alignment
  - *Elevate* residual limb (stump) first 24 hours.
  - Do **NOT** elevate after *48 hours.*
- Provide passive range of motion (ROM).
- Encourage prone position periodically to decrease risk of contracture.
- Proper stump bandaging to prepare for prosthesis
- Coordinate of care with OT, PT, and social worker.
- Assess and address grieving.
- Administer analgesics and antibiotics.
- ✓ REMEMBER: Phantom limb pain is real and requires pharmacological interventions; be sure to assess and address client grief.

Question

Which action by the unlicensed assistive personnel (UAP) requires immediate follow-up by the nurse?

A. Positioning a client who is 12 hours post above-the-knee amputation (AKA) with the residual limb elevated

B. Assisting a client with ambulation while the client uses a cane on the unaffected side

C. Accompanying a client who has lupus erythematosus to sit outside in the sun during a break

D. Helping a client with rheumatoid arthritis to the bathroom after the client takes celecoxib (Celebrex)

Osteoporosis

Risk Factors

- Small-boned postmenopausal females, Caucasian, Asian, pregnancy, breastfeeding, family history
- Diet low in calcium
- Excessive alcohol, tobacco, and caffeine
- Sedentary lifestyle
- Low testosterone level in men
- Diabetes, cirrhosis, corticosteroids, loop diuretics

Symptoms

- Dowager's hump (outward curvature of the upper spine)
- Kyphosis of the dorsal spine
- Loss of height
- Pathological fractures
- Compression fracture of spine can occur

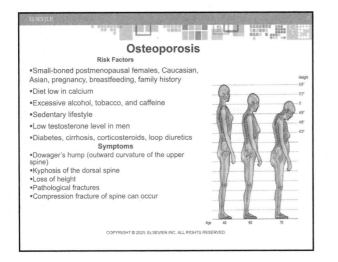

Alendronate: take daily -
fasting ①morning, stay upright

Nursing and Collaborative Management

- Keep bed in low position.
- Provide adequate lighting.
- Avoid using throw rugs.
- Provide assistance with ambulation.
- Follow regular exercise program.
- Encourage diet high in vitamin D, protein, and calcium.
- Encourage 20 minutes of UV exposure a day.
- Routine DEXA screening begins at 60.

Drug Therapy

- **Bisphosphonates**
  ✓ Alendronate, etidronate, zoledronic acid, ibandronate, pamidronate, risedronate
- **Selective Estrogen Receptor Modulators**
  ✓ Raloxifene HCL
  ✓ Teriparatide
- **Recombinant Parathyroid Hormone**
  ✓ Teriparatide

Question

A postmenopausal client with a BMI of 19 has come to the clinic for an annual examination. Which information is most important for the nurse to prepare for this high-risk client?

A. Osteoporosis
B. Obesity
C. Anorexia
D. Breast cancer

Question

The nurse is conducting an osteoporosis screening clinic at a health fair. Which information should the nurse provide to individuals who are at risk for osteoporosis? (Select all that apply.)

A. Limit alcohol and stop smoking
B. Suggest supplementing the diet with vitamin E
C. Promote regular weight-bearing exercise
D. Implement a home safety plan to prevent falls
E. Propose a regular sleep pattern of 8 hours nightly

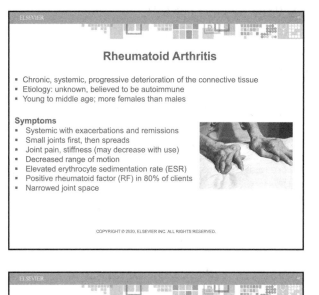

Rheumatoid Arthritis

- Chronic, systemic, progressive deterioration of the connective tissue
- Etiology: unknown, believed to be autoimmune
- Young to middle age; more females than males

Symptoms
- Systemic with exacerbations and remissions
- Small joints first, then spreads
- Joint pain, stiffness (may decrease with use)
- Decreased range of motion
- Elevated erythrocyte sedimentation rate (ESR)
- Positive rheumatoid factor (RF) in 80% of clients
- Narrowed joint space

Nursing and Collaborative Management

Drug Therapy
- High-dose ASA or NSAIDs
- Systemic corticosteroids
- Disease-modifying antirheumatic drugs (DMARDs)
  - Methotrexate
  - Sulfasalazine
  - Hydroxychloroquine
  - Leflunomide
  - Adalimumab

Collaborative Management
- Heat and cold applications
- Weight management
- Rest and joint protection to maintain function
- Use assistive devices
  - ✓ Shower chair
  - ✓ Canes, walkers
  - ✓ Straight-back chairs, elevated seats

Lupus Erythematosus

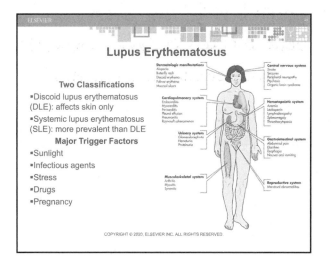

Two Classifications
- Discoid lupus erythematosus (DLE): affects skin only
- Systemic lupus erythematosus (SLE): more prevalent than DLE

Major Trigger Factors
- Sunlight
- Infectious agents
- Stress
- Drugs
- Pregnancy

Stress: marital /prenatal Counseling.

Nursing and Collaborative Management

Nursing Assessment
- ✓ DLE: scaly rash and/or butterfly rash on bridge of nose
- ✓ SLE: joint pain, fever, nephritis, and pericarditis
- ✓ Photosensitivity

Collaborative Management
- ▪ Teaching
- ✓ Drugs
- ✓ Pain management
- ✓ Disease process
- ✓ Conservation of energy
- ✓ Avoid exposure to ultraviolet rays.
- ✓ Avoid/reduce stress.
- ✓ Use mild soaps, creams for skin care.
- ✓ Use steroids for joint inflammation.
- ▪ Therapeutic exercise and heat therapy
- ▪ Pregnancy counseling

★ Pain management

Degenerative Joint Disease (Osteoarthritis)

- ▪ Joint pain increases with activity
- ▪ Morning stiffness
- ▪ Crepitus
- ▪ Limited movement
- ▪ Joint enlargements

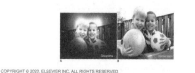

Bone hypertrophy (bone spur)
Cartilage particles
Loss of cartilage

Nursing and Collaborative Management
- ▪ Follow weight-reduction diet
- ▪ Excessive use of involved joint may accelerate degeneration
- ▪ Use proper body mechanics
- ▪ Keep joints in functional position
- ▪ Apply heat and cold applications for pain and stiffness
- ▪ Administer NSAIDs, opioid analgesics, and intraarticular corticosteroids

Opposite side can become
affected: Compensation.

Glaucoma

Primary Open Angle
- ▪ Drainage channels become clogged
- ▪ Aqueous humor flow is reduced in the trabecular meshwork

Primary Closure Angle
- ▪ Bulging lens disrupts flow
- ▪ Silent thief of vision

- ▪ Normally painless until later stages
- ▪ Loss of peripheral vision
- ▪ May see halos around lights
- ▪ Diagnosed with tonometer to measure intraocular pressure

Goal: ↓ IOP — eye drops:
beta-blockers. (∅ pupil impact)
· Avoid straining activities

Nursing and Collaborative Management

Keys to Treatment
- ↓ Intraocular pressure
- ↓ Aqueous humor production
- ↑ Drainage of aqueous humor
- Teach client and family proper eye drop instillation and how to avoid activities that can increase intraocular pressure.

Acute Care for Closure Angle
- Topical cholinergic agent
- Hyperosmotic agent
- Laser peripheral iridotomy
- Surgical iridectomy

Ambulatory/Home Care
- Drug Therapy
  - ✓ β-Adrenergic blockers
  - ✓ α-Adrenergic agonists
  - ✓ Cholinergic agents (miotics)
  - ✓ Carbonic anhydrase inhibitors
- Surgical options
- ALT
- Trabeculectomy

Question

The nurse observes an older client with glaucoma administer eye drops by tilting back the head, instilling each drop close to the inner canthus, and keeping the eye closed for 15 seconds. Which action should the nurse take first?

A. Ask the client whether another family member is available to administer the drops

B. Review the correct steps of the procedure with the client

C. Administer the eye drops correctly in the other eye to demonstrate the technique

D. Discuss the importance of correct eye drop administration for persons with glaucoma

Cataracts

Clouding or opacity of the lens due to trauma, aging, or genetic defect

Early Signs
- Blurred vision
- Decreased color perception

Late Signs
- Double vision
- Clouded pupil

Nursing and Collaborative Management
Preoperative
- Assess current medications
- Stop anticoagulants before surgery
- Teach technique to instill eye drops

Postoperative
- Wear eye shield while sleeping
- Avoid lifting >10 lb
- Avoid lying on operative side
- Report signs of ↑ IOP
- Acute pain is an abnormal finding

Handwritten note: R/t aging: Ideal removal — one eye at a time.

Question

The nurse is teaching an 86-year-old client who has glaucoma and bilateral hearing loss. Which intervention should the nurse implement?

A. Maintain constant eye contact
B. Stand on the side unaffected by glaucoma
C. Speak in a lower tone of voice
D. Keep the environment dimly lit

Eye Trauma/Injury

Trauma
- Determine type of injury
- Early notification of HCP
- Position client in sitting position to reduce intraocular pressure
- Never attempt to remove embedded object
- Irrigate eye if a chemical injury has occurred

Detached Retina
- Described as curtain falling over visual field
- Painless with sudden loss of vision
- May see black spots or floaters (indicates bleeding has occurred with detachment)
- Retina repaired surgically
- Keep eye patch over affected area

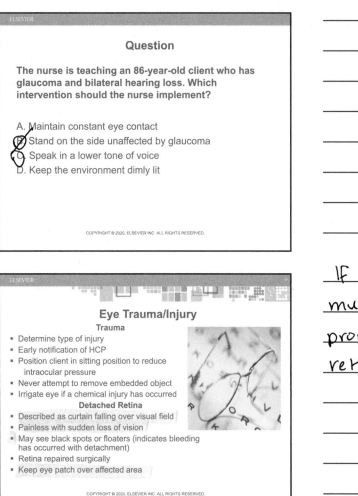

If air bubble in place: head must be kept down, or lay prone: 20hr (1 wk) to keep retina attached.

Hearing Loss

Conductive Hearing Loss
- Sounds do not travel to the inner ear
- May benefit from hearing aid
- Cerumen buildup

Sensorineural Hearing Loss
- Sound distorted by defect in inner ear

Common Causes
- Infections
- Ototoxic drugs
- ✓Gentamicin
- ✓Vancomycin
- ✓Lasix
- Trauma
- Aging process

Symptoms
- Inability to hear whisper from 1 to 2 feet
- Shouting in conversations
- Turning head to favor one ear
- Loud volume on TV

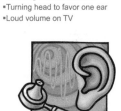

Nursing and Collaborative Management

- Face the client directly when speaking.
- Ensure the client is wearing hearing aids and eyeglasses, if appropriate.
- Speak at a normal tone being sure to enunciate words.
- Rephrase questions instead of repeating them.
- Do not cover mouth with hand when speaking.

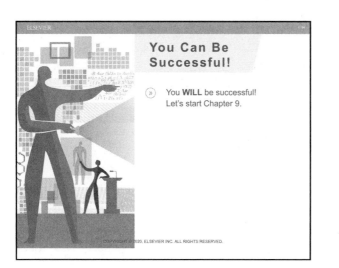

You Can Be Successful!

You **WILL** be successful!
Let's start Chapter 9.

Weber: Sensorineural

Chapter **8** **Movement, Coordination, and Sensory Input** **139**

9 Pediatric Nursing

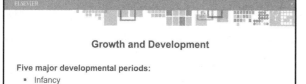

Growth and Development

Five major developmental periods:
- Infancy
- Toddler
- Preschool
- School age
- Adolescence

Developmental theories most widely used in explaining child growth and development:
- Freud's psychosexual stages
- Erikson's stages of psychosocial development
- Piaget's stages of cognitive development
- Kohlberg's stages of moral development

Question

The nurse directs the unlicensed assistive personnel (UAP) to play with a 4-year-old child on bed rest. Which activities should the nurse recommend? (Select all that apply.)

A. Monopoly board game
B. Checkers
C. 50-piece puzzle
D. Hand puppets
E. Coloring book

Question

While receiving IV antibiotics for sepsis, a 2-month-old infant is crying inconsolably, despite the parent's presence. The nurse recognizes that the infant is exhibiting symptoms related to which likely condition?

A. Allergic reaction to antibiotics
B. Pain related to IV infiltration
C. Separation anxiety from parent
D. Hunger and thirst

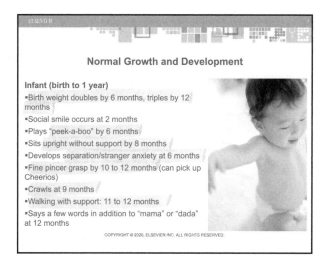

Normal Growth and Development

Infant (birth to 1 year)

- Birth weight doubles by 6 months, triples by 12 months
- Social smile occurs at 2 months
- Plays "peek-a-boo" by 6 months
- Sits upright without support by 8 months
- Develops separation/stranger anxiety at 6 months
- Fine pincer grasp by 10 to 12 months (can pick up Cheerios)
- Crawls at 9 months
- Walking with support: 11 to 12 months
- Says a few words in addition to "mama" or "dada" at 12 months

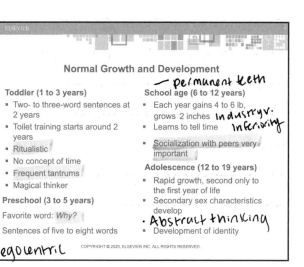

Normal Growth and Development

Toddler (1 to 3 years)

- Two- to three-word sentences at 2 years
- Toilet training starts around 2 years
- Ritualistic
- No concept of time
- Frequent tantrums
- Magical thinker

Preschool (3 to 5 years)

Favorite word: *Why?*

Sentences of five to eight words

egocentric

School age (6 to 12 years)

— permanent teeth

- Each year gains 4 to 6 lb, grows 2 inches — *Industry v.*
- Learns to tell time — *Inferiority*
- Socialization with peers very important

Adolescence (12 to 19 years)

- Rapid growth, second only to the first year of life
- Secondary sex characteristics develop
- *Abstract thinking*
- Development of identity

Pain Assessment and Management

- Assessment is based on verbal and nonverbal cues from child and includes parents' information.
- Be aware of developmental responses.
- Use appropriate pain scale.
- Safety is a major priority for administering medication.
- Make sure dose is *safe for age and weight.*

Nonpharmacological Interventions
- **Infants** may respond best to pacifiers, holding, and rocking.
- **Toddlers** and preschoolers may respond best to distraction.
- **School-age children** and adolescents may use guided imagery.

Pharmacological Interventions
- Verify that the prescribed dose is safe based on weight.
- Monitor the child's vital signs after administration of opioids.
- Children as young as 5 years of age may be taught to use a client-controlled analgesia (PCA) pump.

Handwritten notes:

Birth length: ↑ by 50% by 12 mo.

Steady head control at 4 mo.
- 10 mo window: choking concern

Moro: Startle reflex — disappear 4 mo. Dx: cerebral palsy.

Infant: Solitary play: 1) Risk of choking/strangulation.

Infancy: Trust v. Mistrust for hope establishment.

18 mo: Throw ball overhead

24 mo: Kick a ball / tip toes

20 baby teeth: dental hygiene

2: Feed from spoon / drink from a cup.

Toddler: ∅ Concept of time
↓
magical thinking: parallel play

Preschool: 5 lb weight gain / year
2 1/3 - 3 in / year. 4y: birth length doubled. Visual acuity 20/20.
3y / tricycle   4y / scissors

Preschool → group play. Initiative v. Guilt (w/ purpose).

- Adolescence: Risk takers, Identity v. Role confusion.

Poisonings

- Frequent cause of childhood injury—teach poison-proofing methods for the home
- Children <6 years with peak at 2 years of age
- GI disturbance is a common symptom
- Burns of mouth and pharynx with caustic poisonings
- Identify poisonous agent quickly
- Check ABCs
- Teach parents NOT to make the child vomit because it may cause more damage
- Call Poison Control Center or 911, based on how the child is acting

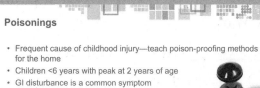

Immunizations

- Common cold *does not* contraindicate immunization unless the fever is >37.2° C (99° F) 101°F
- A fever <38.9° C (<102° F) and redness and soreness at the injection site are normal for 2 to 3 days after vaccination.
- Call healthcare provider (HCP) if child has high-pitched crying, seizures, or high fever.
- Use acetaminophen orally, before and every 4 to 6 hours after for 24 hours.
- Hold MMR vaccine if anaphylactic reaction to neomycin/eggs.

*Consolobility to ↓ trauma
· Acetaminophen: temp management to prevent febrile seizures.
· Allergy to bakers yeast: ∅ hep B. vaccine.
MMR / varicella: Same day or 28 days between.

Question

A parent is preparing a **5-year-old** child for kindergarten. The child has not received any immunizations. Which vaccines should be given to this child? (Select all that apply.)

(A) DTaP
(B) Inactivated polio virus (IVP)
(C) Varicella
D. Pneumococcal conjugate vaccine (PCV)
E. Trivalent inactivated influenza vaccine (TIV)

ELSEVIER

Question

Which vaccines should the nurse expect to be prescribed for a 2-month-old brought into the pediatrician's office for a well-baby checkup? (Select all that apply.)

A. DTaP
B. Hep B
C. Hep C
D. HIB
E. IPV
F. PCV

CDC: milestone tracker
· vaccines / milestones

ELSEVIER

Communicable Diseases

The incidence of common childhood communicable diseases has declined greatly since the advent of immunizations, but they do occur, and nurses should be able to identify the infection.

- Measles
- Rubeola
- Rubella
- Roseola
- Mumps
- Pertussis
- Diphtheria
- Varicella
- Erythema infectiosum (fifth disease)

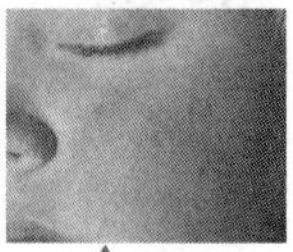

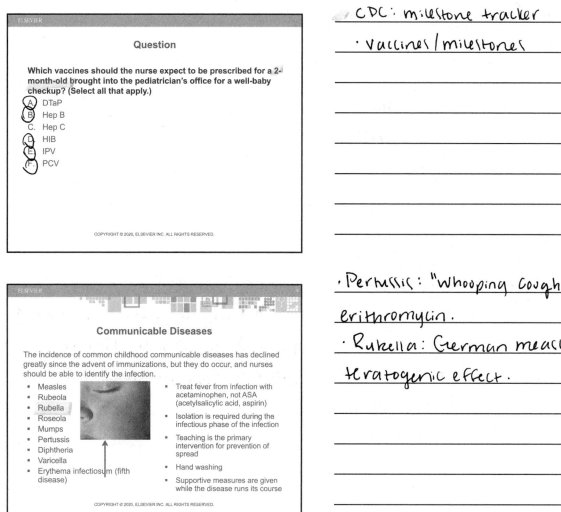

- Treat fever from infection with acetaminophen, not ASA (acetylsalicylic acid, aspirin)
- Isolation is required during the infectious phase of the infection
- Teaching is the primary intervention for prevention of spread
- Hand washing
- Supportive measures are given while the disease runs its course

· Pertussis: "whooping cough" — Tx: erithromycin.
· Rubella: German measles — teratogenic effect.

ELSEVIER

Respiratory Disorders

- Be familiar with normal values for respiratory and pulse rates for children.
- **Cardinal signs of respiratory distress:**
  - Restlessness
  - Increased respiratory rate
  - Increased pulse rate
  - Diaphoresis
- Respiratory failure usually occurs before cardiac failure.

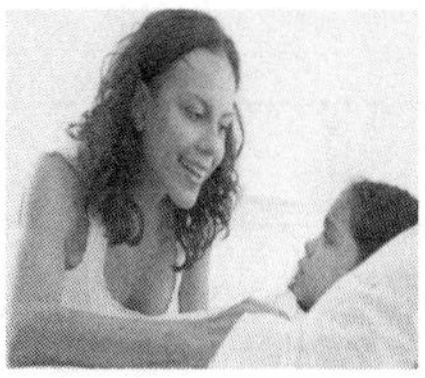

Respiratory Disorders

- Nasopharyngitis/tonsillitis
- Otitis media
- Bronchitis
- RSV
- Epiglottitis
- Croup
- Asthma
- Cystic fibrosis

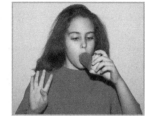

Respiratory Disorders

Nasopharyngitis/Tonsillitis

- May be viral or bacterial
- Treatment important if related to streptococcal infection
- Check prothrombin time (PT) and partial thromboplastin time (PTT) before surgery
- Monitor for bleeding
- Highest risk for bleeding is during first 24 hours and 5 to 10 days postoperative

Otitis Media

- Fever, pulling at ear, discharge
- Administer antibiotics
- Position on affected side
- Reduce temperature to prevent seizures

Bronchitis

- Inflammation of trachea and bronchi
- Rhinitis and cough
- Crackles and rhonchi
- Symptomatic treatment

Question

The nurse is caring for a child who had a tonsillectomy 2 hours ago. Which sign or symptom most likely relates to a complication?

A. Apical rate 90 beats/min
B. Blood pressure 96/50
C. Frequent swallowing
D. Nasal congestion

Handwritten note:
Otitis Media: ↑ fever : need good temp control. If ∅ tubes: place affected side. If tubes, place on opposite side.

S/S:
Epiglottis: tongue out, drooling,
protruded chin, tripod position.

Respiratory Disorders

Respiratory syncytial virus bronchiolitis (RSV)
- Isolate the child (contact isolation)
- Monitor respiratory status
- Maintain patent airway
- Antiviral agent (ribavirin aerosols)
- RSV prophylaxis with monoclonal antibody palivizumab (Synagis) in high-risk children <2 years of age

Epiglottitis
- Major cause is HIB
- Fever, sore throat, muffled voice, drooling
- IV antibiotics
- Do NOT examine the throat
- Prepare for tracheostomy

Croup
- Primarily viral infection
- Hoarseness, brassy or barky cough; respiratory distress; worse at night
- Supportive measures
  - ✓ Cool mist humidity
  - ✓ Increased oral intake
  - ✓ Oral dexamethasone

Question

A 4-year-old is brought to the clinic with a fever of 103° F, sore throat, and moderate respiratory distress caused by a suspected bacterial infection. Which medical diagnosis is a contraindication to obtaining a throat culture in the child?

- A. Tonsillitis
- B. Streptococcal infection
- C. Bronchiolitis
- D. Epiglottitis

Question

The nurse is caring for a 2-year-old child suspected of having croup. Which early sign of respiratory distress requires the nurse's immediate attention?

A. Cyanosis
B. Restlessness
C. Crying
D. Barking cough

Asthma: The Leading Cause of Chronic Illness in Children

Allergies influence persistence and severity of the illness

Complex disorder involving biochemical, immunologic, infections, endocrine, and psychological factors

Nursing and Collaborative Management

- S/S: tight cough, expiratory wheezing, decreased peak flow levels
- Monitor for respiratory distress, need for O$_2$ nebulizer therapy

- Rescue versus maintenance medications
- Evaluate effects of β-adrenergic agonists, such as albuterol and levalbuterol, as well as corticosteroids

---

Question

The nurse is reinforcing teaching for a school-age child and the child's parent regarding the administration of inhaled beclomethasone dipropionate and albuterol for the treatment of asthma. Which statement by the parent indicates that teaching has been effective?

A. "I'll keep the inhalers in the refrigerator."

B. "My child only needs to use inhalers when the peak flow numbers are in the red."

C. "My child will take the bronchodilator first, then the corticosteroid."

D. "My child will take the corticosteroid first, wait a few minutes, and then take the bronchodilator."

Cystic Fibrosis (CF)

- Most frequently occurring inherited disease of Caucasian children
- Transmitted by an autosomal recessive gene
- Chronic multisystem disorder
- Abnormally thick mucus
- Primarily lung and pancreatic involvement
- + Newborn screening test

- First sign may be meconium ileus at birth
- High sweat chloride concentration (pilocarpine test or sweat test)
- Delayed growth, poor weight gain
- Pancreatic enzymes with each meal and snacks, fat-soluble vitamins
- Teach family percussion and postural drainage techniques

Handwritten note:
- Common: delayed growth ↑ caloric needs.

Question

The nurse is reinforcing discharge teaching for parents of a 4-year-old with cystic fibrosis. Which statement by the parents demonstrates understanding of the teaching presented?

A. "We will discourage our child from playing outdoors."

B. "We will use pancreatic enzymes only if needed."

C. "We will thoroughly wash our child's hands after toileting."

D. "We will schedule a physical therapist evaluation."

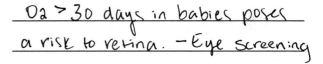

Cardiovascular Disorders: Congenital Heart Disorders

- May be classified as acyanotic or cyanotic. Most important is the management of the symptoms. For descriptions and illustrations of congenital cardiovascular disorders, see a textbook or an NCLEX review manual:

- *Evolve Reach Comprehensive Review for the NCLEX-RN Examination* (powered by HESI)

- *Mosby's Comprehensive Review of Nursing for the NCLEX-RN Examination*

- *Saunders Comprehensive Review for the NCLEX-RN Examination Nursing and Collaborative Management*

Cardiovascular Disorders: Heart Failure

- Common complication of congenital heart disorders

- S/S: pedal edema, neck vein distention, respiratory distress, fatigue, irritability, sudden weight gain

- Monitor vital signs, elevate head of bed, O_2.

- Digoxin, diuretics, and ACE inhibitors

- Weigh daily on same scale

- Maintain nutritional status; feeding should not last >30 minutes

- Plan frequent rest periods

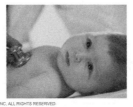

Handwritten note: O_2 > 30 days in babies poses a risk to retina. — Eye screening

Managing Digoxin Therapy in Children

- Count apical rate when child is at rest; withhold medication if pulse is <90 to 110 beats/min in infants or <70 beats/min in older children.
- Notify healthcare provider.
- Do not skip or try to make up doses.
- Give 1 to 2 hours before meals.
- Watch for S/S of toxicity and teach them to parents: vomiting, anorexia, diarrhea, muscle weakness, drowsiness.
- Provide adequate potassium in the diet.

Handwritten notes:

0.5-2: normal digoxin toxicity
Antidote: digivind
↓ K⁺ levels: ↑ risk of toxicity

Rheumatic Fever

- Peaks in school-age children
- Most common cause of acquired heart disease
- Affects connective tissue
- S/S: sore throat that appears to be improving, then fever develops along with rash, chorea, elevated erythrocyte sedimentation rate
- Antibiotic prophylaxis for invasive procedures

Nursing and Collaborative Management

- Encourage compliance with drug regimens
- Penicillin remains the drug of choice
- Salicylates are used to control the inflammatory process and to reduce fever and discomfort
- Prednisone may be indicated in some patients with heart failure
- Bed rest or at least limited activity during the acute illness
- Provide emotional support

Handwritten notes:

Chorea: involuntary jerking
Concern: ♡ valves
ABX: penicillin, 2 mo tx
Strep → progresses →
Sore throat, rheumatic fever.

Question

A 2-year-old child's blood work is evaluated by the nurse. Considering that the child is prescribed furosemide, captopril, and digoxin for congestive heart failure, which value should the nurse verify with the laboratory?

A. Hypocalcemia
B. Hypernatremia
C. Low hemoglobin
D. Hypokalemia

Question

A pediatric client is prescribed digoxin for a congenital heart defect. The maintenance dosage ordered is 50 mcg/kg/day. The child weighs 10 kg. The prescription requires the digoxin to be administered twice daily. The nurse prepares _____ mcg of digoxin at each dose.

Question

The nurse reviews the medication record of a 2-month-old and notes that the infant was given a scheduled dose of digoxin with a documented apical pulse of 76 beats/min. Which action should the nurse take first?

A. Assess the current apical pulse rate

B. Observe for the onset of diarrhea

C. Complete an adverse occurrence report

D. Determine the serum potassium level

Kawasaki Disease

- Acute systemic vasculitis
- Occurs in children <5 years
- Self-limiting disease
- 25% of children develop coronary artery dilation or aneurysm if left untreated.
- Symptoms: fever >5 days, erythema of palms and soles, peeling of hands and feet, bilateral conjunctival inflammation without exudate, erythema of lips, oropharynx, strawberry tongue, rash, and cervical lymphadenopathy
- Nursing and collaborative management
  - Compliance with medication
    - High-dose IVIG
    - Aspirin
    - Possible anticoagulation therapy

Handwritten notes:

50 mcg (10 kg) / day
500 / day
250 mcg dose

★ Strawberry tongue

Down Syndrome

- Flat, broad nasal bridge; upward, outward-slanting eyes
- Commonly associated problems:
  - Cardiac defects
  - Delayed development
  - Respiratory infections
- Always evaluate functional age
- Feed to back and side of mouth due to tongue thrust
- Support child/parent relationship to achieve highest level of functioning
- Refer family to early intervention program

Question

The nurse is caring for a 16-year-old client with Down syndrome who has a mental age of 5. Which priority nursing action should be included in this client's plan of care?

A. Monitoring for hearing loss
B. Monitoring I&O
C. Providing a dependable routine
D. Providing small puzzles

Cerebral Palsy (CP)

Diagnosis
- Made on evaluation of child
- Permanent injury to the motor centers of the brain before, during, or after birth
- Persistent neonatal reflexes after 6 months—no parachute reflex
- Spasticity, muscle, and motor tone abnormalities

Nursing and Collaborative Management
- Prevent aspiration with feedings
- Medication for seizures, muscle spasticity, muscle pain

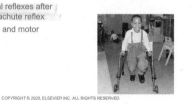

Consults:
Speech, nutrition, OT, PT

Commonly seen: premature
birth or anoxic event during
★ Risk of falling
· Muscle spasms meds.

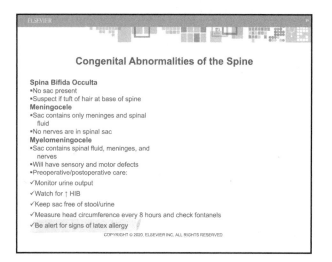

Congenital Abnormalities of the Spine

Spina Bifida Occulta
- No sac present
- Suspect if tuft of hair at base of spine

Meningocele
- Sac contains only meninges and spinal fluid
- No nerves are in spinal sac

Myelomeningocele
- Sac contains spinal fluid, meninges, and nerves
- Will have sensory and motor defects
- Preoperative/postoperative care:
- ✓ Monitor urine output
- ✓ Watch for ↑ HIB
- ✓ Keep sac free of stool/urine
- ✓ Measure head circumference every 8 hours and check fontanels
- ✓ Be alert for signs of latex allergy

Myelomeningocele: risk of retaining urine in bladder.

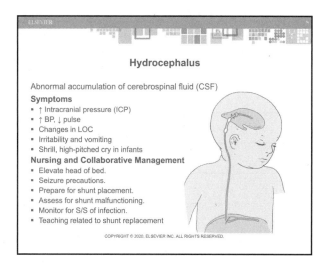

Hydrocephalus

Abnormal accumulation of cerebrospinal fluid (CSF)

Symptoms
- ↑ Intracranial pressure (ICP)
- ↑ BP, ↓ pulse
- Changes in LOC
- Irritability and vomiting
- Shrill, high-pitched cry in infants

Nursing and Collaborative Management
- Elevate head of bed.
- Seizure precautions.
- Prepare for shunt placement.
- Assess for shunt malfunctioning.
- Monitor for S/S of infection.
- Teaching related to shunt replacement

headache, spontaneous vomiting may come before change in LOC when ↑ICP.

Question

A child with hydrocephalus is 1 day postoperative for revision of a ventriculoatrial shunt. Which finding is most important for the nurse to assess first?

A. Increased blood pressure
B. Increased temperature
C. Increased serum glucose
D. Increased hematocrit

Seizures/Epilepsy

- Uncontrolled neuronal electrical activity
- More common in children younger than 2 years

Types of Seizures
Generalized

- Tonic/clonic (formerly grand mal)
- Aura
- Loss of consciousness
- Tonic phase: stiffness of body
- Clonic phase: spasms and relaxation
- Postictal phase: sleepy and disoriented

Myoclonic

- Sudden, brief contraction of muscle, group of muscles

Partial Seizures

- Specific area in the brain; limited symptoms

Absence Seizures (formerly petit mal)

- Momentary loss of consciousness, appears to be daydreaming, poor performance in school
- Lasts 5 to 30 seconds

Status Epilepticus

- Series of seizures at intervals too brief to allow the child to regain consciousness

Seizures: Nursing and Collaborative Management

- Maintain patent airway
- Side rails up/pad side rails
- Do not use tongue blade
- Administer anticonvulsants

Phenobarbital and Primidone

- Generalized tonic clonic
- Partial
- Status epilepticus

Phenytoin

- Generalized tonic clonic
- Partial
- Status epilepticus

Carbamazepine

- Generalized tonic clonic
- Partial

Fosphenytoin (IM, IV)

- Generalized status epilepticus
- Treatment of seizures during nuerosurgery
- Short-term parenteral replacement for oral phenytoin

Valproic acid

- Generalized tonic clonic
- Absence
- Myoclonic
- Partial

Clonazepam

- Absence
- Myoclonic
- Infantile spasms
- Partial

Question

The nurse observes an adolescent client experiencing a tonic-clonic seizure. Which intervention should the nurse provide first?

A. Restrain the client to protect against injury
B. Flex the neck to ensure stabilization
C. Use a tongue blade to open the airway
D. Turn client on side to aid ventilation

Question

The healthcare provider prescribes the anticonvulsant phenytoin for an adolescent with a seizure disorder. The nurse should instruct the client to notify the healthcare provider if which condition develops?

A. Dry mouth
B. Dizziness
C. Sore throat
D. Gingival hyperplasia

Bacterial Meningitis

Usually caused by *Haemophilus influenzae* type B, *Streptococcus pneumoniae*, and *Neisseria meningitidis*

Diagnostic procedures include lumbar puncture for laboratory analysis

Signs and Symptoms

- Petechial or purpuric rashes, especially when associated with shock-like state
- Older children: include S/S of increased ICP, neck stiffness, + Kernig's sign, + Brudzinski's sign
- Infants: classic signs absent; poor feeding, vomiting, irritability, bulging fontanels

Nursing and Collaborative Management

- Isolate at least 24 hours
- Administer antibiotics
- Frequent VS and neurological checks
- Increased ICP, muscle twitching, and changes in LOC
- Measure head circumference daily.
- SIADH (syndrome of inappropriate antidiuretic hormone) occurs frequently
- Fluid restriction may be necessary

Handwritten note: ★ Nuchal rigidity Tx: penicillins

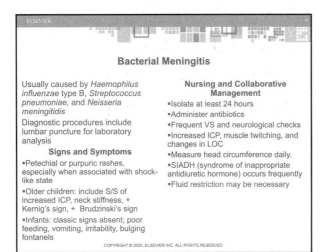

Reye Syndrome and Muscular Dystrophy

Reye Syndrome

- Etiology often, but *not always*, associated with aspirin use and influenza or varicella
- Rapidly progressing encephalopathy; altered hepatic function
- S/S: lethargy progressing to coma, vomiting, hypoglycemia
- Neurological checks, maintain airway
- Mannitol for ICP control
- Early diagnosis is important to improve client outcome

Duchenne Muscular Dystrophy

- Onset ages 2 to 6 yr
- Most severe and most common MD
- X-linked recessive disorder

Diagnosis

- Muscle biopsy
- Serum creatine phosphokinase (CK)

Symptoms

- Delayed walking and frequent falls
- Gower sign
- Easily tires when walking

Interventions

- Exercise and assistive devices for ambulation
- Prevent falls (loss of ambulation at 8 to 12 years of age)

Handwritten note: • Reye Syndrome: maintain an airway.
Gower sign: scissoring of legs until fully upright.

Renal Disorders

Urinary Tract Infection (UTI)

More common with female anatomy

Symptoms
- Poor food intake
- Strong-smelling urine
- Fever
- Pain with urination

Nursing and Collaborative Management
- Obtain urine culture before starting antibiotics.
- Teach home care.
  - ✓ Finish all antibiotics.
  - ✓ Avoid bubble baths.
  - ✓ Increase intake of acidic fluids, such as apple or cranberry juice.

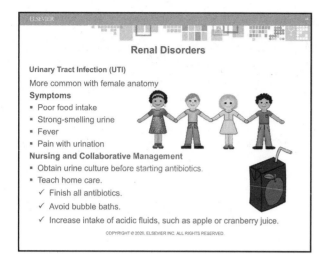

Acute Glomerulonephritis (AGN)

Common Features
- Oliguria, hematuria, proteinuria
- Edema
- Hypertension
- Circulatory congestion

Therapeutic Management
- Maintenance of fluid balance
- Treatment of hypertension

Nursing Assessment
- Recent strep infection
- Dark "iced tea" urine
- Irritable and/or lethargic

Nursing and Collaborative Management
- VS every 4 hours
- Daily weights
- Low-sodium, low-potassium diet

Strep infection in kidney blocks GFR. GFR ↓
- tea-colored urine
- diuretics w/ no response — no output.
- ↑BP

Nephrotic Syndrome

Characterized by increased glomerular permeability to protein

Assessment
- Frothy urine
- Massive proteinuria
- Edema
- Anorexia

Nursing and Collaborative Management
- Reducing excretion of protein
- Reducing or preventing fluid retention
- Preventing infection
- Skin care
- Administer medications.
- Diuretics, corticosteroid therapy, immunosuppressants, antibiotics
- Small frequent feeding

Discharge Teaching
- Daily weights
- Side effects of meds
- Prevent infections

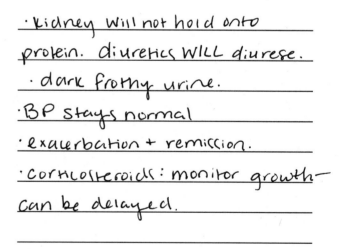

- kidney will not hold onto protein. diuretics WILL diurese.
- dark frothy urine.
- BP stays normal
- exacerbation + remission.
- corticosteroids: monitor growth — can be delayed.

Question

A school-age child with nephrotic syndrome is seen at the clinic 2 days after discharge from the hospital. Which assessment is most important for the nurse to perform after discharge?

A. Pain
B. Capillary refill
C. Urine ketones
D. Daily weight

Question

A 3-week-old infant with pyloric stenosis has severe vomiting. Which signs of dehydration should the nurse anticipate in the infant? (Select all that apply.)

A. Sunken fontanel
B. Increased urine output
C. High serum hematocrit level
D. Cracked lips
E. Thirst

Diarrhea

Worldwide, leading cause of death in children <5 years of age

- Classified as acute or chronic
- Common problem for infants

Assessment
- Depressed/sunken eyes
- Weight loss
- ↓ Urine output

Nursing and Collaborative Management
- Fluid and electrolyte balance
- Rehydration
- Maintenance fluid therapy
- Reintroduction of adequate diet
- Do not give antidiarrheal agents

· Rotovirus can be a cause

Gastrointestinal Disorders

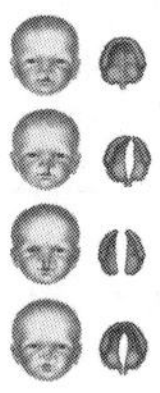

Cleft Lip or Cleft Palate
- Malformation of the face or oral cavity
- Initial closure of cleft lip is performed when infant is approximately 3 months
- Closure of cleft palate at around 9 to 15 months
- Promote bonding
- Breck/Haberman feeder and slow-flow nipple
- Maintain airway
- No straws or spoons, only soft foods for cleft palate

Pyloric Stenosis
- Common in first-born males
- Vomiting becomes projectile around day 14 after birth
- Dehydration, weight loss, and failure to thrive

Intussusception
- Telescoping of one part of intestine
- Emergency intervention is needed
- Sudden onset of crampy abdominal pain, inconsolable crying, and drawing knees to chest in otherwise healthy child

---

Hematological Disorders

Sickle Cell Anemia
- Autosomal recessive disorder
- Fetal Hgb does not sickle

Maintenance
- Keep well hydrated
- Do not give supplemental iron
- Give folic acid orally
- PCN prophylactically at 2 months of age

Crisis: Fever and Pain
- Bed rest, hydration, and analgesia
- Improve oxygen utilization
- Blood replacement and antibiotic therapy

Hemophilia
- X-linked recessive disorder
- Factor VIII deficiency

Interventions
- Administer fresh frozen plasma
- Apply pressure to even minor bleeds because of increased risk for bleeding

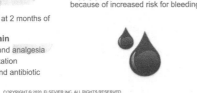

Question

A child admitted with sickle cell crisis is anemic and has painful joints and a fever of 101° F. Which priority intervention should the nurse include in the plan of care for this child?

A. Maintain oral fluids for hydration
B. Apply cold packs to painful joints
C. Administer aspirin daily for pain and fever
D. Perform range-of-motion exercises to decrease joint pain

Handwritten notes:

- By 12 mo prevents speech impediment.
- Pyloric Stenosis: hypertrophy of pyloric sphincter. Asx: nodule in RUQ. ↓ pressure on sphincter.
- Intussusception: Medical emergency! S/s: PAIN
- Currant colored stool

- Hgb replaced w/ HgbS: ∅ sickle
- Need folic acid for anemia

Lacking clotting factor.

Handwritten notes (top right)

- Build up of PKU can lead to mental retardation.
- Diet maintained until brain is fully developed. Pregnancy - remain diet.

Handwritten note (middle right)

Clicking of hip

Handwritten note (lower right)

- Earlier identification is best: use of brace.

Slide 1

Metabolic and Endocrine Disorders

Phenylketonuria (PKU)

- Autosomal recessive disorder
- Newborn screening (after 24 hours of age)
- Strict adherence to low-phenylalanine diet; prevents mental retardation
- ✓ Special PKU formula
- ✓ Avoid meat, milk, dairy, and aspartame-containing foods
- ✓ Diet: fruits, juices, cereal, bread, and starches

Diabetes
See Chapter 7.

Slide 2

Skeletal Disorders

Fractures
- Visible signs of fractures
- Obtain baseline pulses, color, movement, sensation, temperature, swelling, and pain
- Report any changes immediately

Traction (Fractures not easily reduced by casting and for presurgical stabilization)
- Buck's traction: knee immobilization
- Russell traction: femur/lower leg fracture
- 90 degree/90 degree traction
- Can be skeletal or skin
- Pinned for desired line of pull and flexion at hip and knee of 90 degrees
- Appropriate toys, cast care, prevent cast soilage, monitor NV signs

Congenital Dislocated Hip

Assessment
- Positive Ortolani sign
- Unequal fold of skin on buttocks
- Limited abduction of hip

Nursing and Collaborative Management
- Pavlik harness (worn 24 h/day)
- Surgical correction
- Hip spica cast care

Slide 3

Scoliosis

- S-shaped curvature of the spine
- Most common nontraumatic skeletal condition in children
- Milwaukee brace
- Scoliosis affects both genders at any age, but it is most commonly seen in adolescents

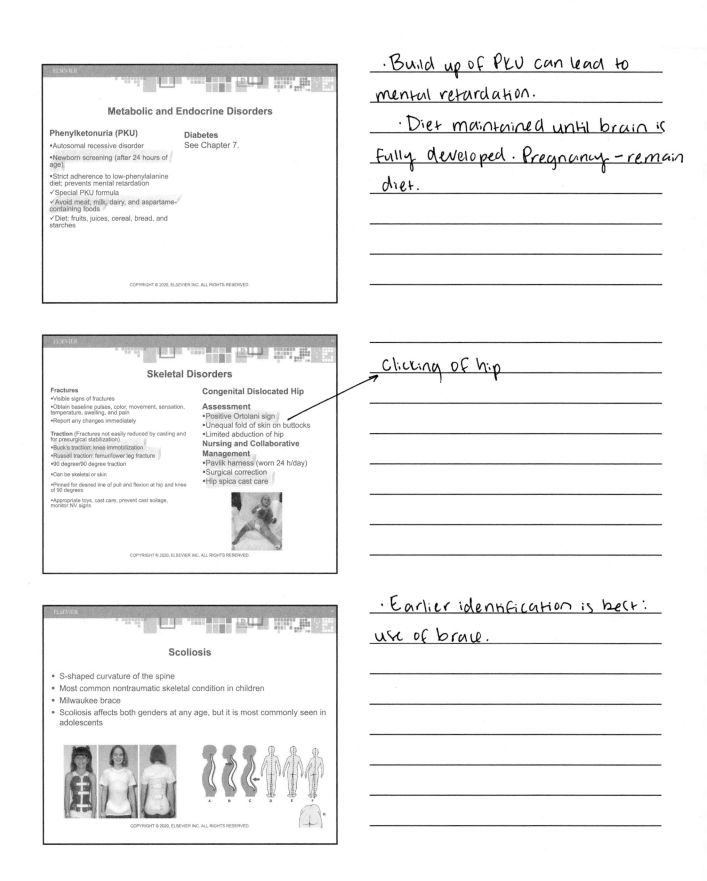

Juvenile Idiopathic Arthritis (JIA)

- Also known as juvenile rheumatoid arthritis (JRA)
- Most common arthritic condition of childhood
- Inflammatory disease involves the joints, connective tissues, and viscera
- Exact cause is unknown, but infections and an autoimmune response have been implicated
- Therapy consists of administration of medications, such as NSAIDs, methotrexate, or aspirin, along with exercise, heat application, and support of joints

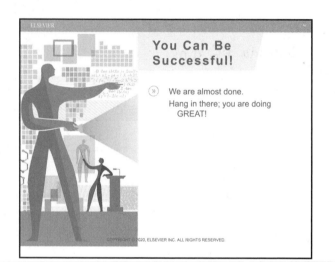

You Can Be Successful!

» We are almost done. Hang in there; you are doing GREAT!

Maternal-Newborn Nursing

Pregnancy

Assess for Intimate Partner Violence (IPV)
- Battering and emotional or physical abuse often begins with pregnancy
- Assess for abuse in private, away from partner
- The nurse needs to know:
  - ✓ Local resources
  - ✓ Where to recommend safety for client

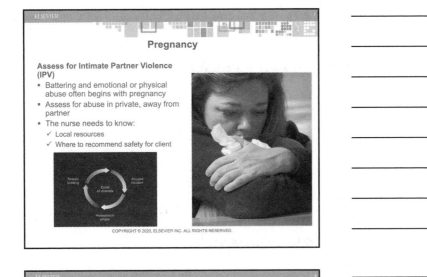

Pregnancy

Gravidity and Parity
Gravida and parity: counts pregnancies, not offspring
- ✓ **Gravida:** number of times a female has been pregnant, regardless of outcome
- ✓ **Para:** number of deliveries (not children) occurred after 20 weeks' gestation
- Multiple births count as one
- Pregnancy loss before 20 weeks counted as abortion but add 1 to gravidity
- Fetal demise after 20 weeks added to parity

Past and Future
GTPAL represents obstetric history:
- **G** = Gravidity (total number of pregnancies)
- **T** = Term pregnancies (after 37 weeks)
- **P** = Preterm pregnancies (before 37 weeks)
- **A** = Abortions (elective or spontaneous): loss before 20 weeks
- **L** = Living children

Pregnancy

Gestation
- Naegele's Rule
- ✓ Count back 3 months from date of last normal menstrual period
- ✓ Add 1 year and 7 days

Fundal Height
- 12 to 13 weeks: fundus rises out of symphysis
- 20 weeks: fundus at umbilicus
- 24 to about 36 weeks: fundal height (in centimeters) from the symphysis is equal to number of weeks of gestation if this is a single pregnancy

Weight gain (Optimal weight gain depends on maternal and fetal factors.)

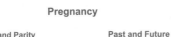

First-trimester average total weight gain is 1 to 2 kg
Approximately 0.5 kg per week for a woman of normal weight during second and third trimesters

Chapter **10** **Maternal-Newborn Nursing** 159

Maternal Psychological Changes

Ambivalence	Occurs early in pregnancy, even with a planned pregnancy
Acceptance	Occurs with the woman's readiness for the experience. Prolonged nonacceptance is a warning sign not directly related to nonacceptance of the child.
Emotional lability	Rapid, unpredictable changes in mood

→ Seen~12-13 wks

Warning Signs of Physical Maternal Changes

1. Abdominal pain/cramping or pelvic pain
2. Decreased or absent fetal movement
3. Fever or chills
4. Urinary symptoms
5. Signs or symptoms of preterm labor
6. Signs of hypertensive disorders

Any infection during pregnancy poses concern!

Common Diagnostic Tests

Maternal
- Urine screen
- Glucose tolerance test
- Uterine activity

Fetal
- Quad screen includes alpha fetoprotein, human chorionic gonadotropin (hCG), estriol, inhibin A; for high-risk pregnancy, chromosomal abnormalities and neural tube defects
- Chorionic villi sampling (CVS) for genetic and chromosomal disorders at 8 to 12 weeks; full bladder required; Rh-negative mother requires RhoGAM (Rh₀[D] immune globulin) postprocedure.

Fetal
- Amniocentesis performed at 16 weeks to determine genetic disorders, at 30 weeks to determine lung maturity; bladder emptied if performed after 20 weeks' gestation; Rh-negative mother requires RhoGAM postprocedure
- Ultrasound: multiple purposes; client must have a full bladder
- Nonstress test (NST) via ultrasound transducer records fetal movement and heart rate after 28 weeks; increase in heart rate (reactivity) expected in healthy fetus
- Biophysical profile (via ultrasound): includes NST results, amniotic fluid volume, fetal breathing movements, fetal tone and body movements
- Uterine activity

Glucose tolerance: 20-24 wks testing.

· Testing: before 20 wks: push fluids for full bladder. Past 20 wks: empty bladder.

Question

A client who is at 36 weeks' gestation is placed in the lithotomy position when she suddenly complains of feeling breathless and light-headed and shows marked pallor. Which action should the nurse take first?

A. Turn the client to a lateral position
B. Place the client in Trendelenburg position
C. Obtain vital signs and pulse oximetry reading
D. Initiate distraction techniques

Question

A client's suspected pregnancy is confirmed. The client tells the nurse that she had three previous pregnancies where she delivered one infant at 39 weeks, twins at 34 weeks, and another infant at 35 weeks. Using the GTPAL notation, how should the nurse record the client's gravidity and parity?

A. 3-0-3-0-3
B. 3-1-1-1-3
C. 4-1-2-0-4
D. 4-2-1-0-3

Labor

True labor
- Pain in lower back radiating to the abdomen
- Regular, rhythmic contractions
- Increased intensity with ambulation
- Progressive cervical dilation and effacement

False labor
- Discomfort localized to the abdomen
- No lower back pain
- Contractions often stop with ambulation or position change

Stages of Labor

First stage: dilation and effacement with 100% cervical effacement and complete dilation of cervix (10 cm). Duration is from 8 to 20 hours in the primipara and 5 to 14 hours in the multipara. Includes 3 phases: latent (0 to 3 cm), active (4 to 7 cm), and transition (8 to 10 cm).

Second stage: begins with complete cervical dilatation; expulsion ending with birth of the baby. Generally lasts from a few minutes to 2 hours.

Third stage: placental separation. It begins with the birth of the baby and ends with the expulsion of the placenta. This process can last up to 30 minutes, with an average length of 5 to 10 minutes.

Fourth stage: defined as the first 1 to 4 hours after delivery of the placenta. Monitor for excessive bleeding and uterine atony.

Labor Progression

- **Cervical dilation:** stretching of the cervical os to allow passage of the infant (from 0 to 10 cm)
- **Effacement:** thinning and shortening of the cervix (0% to 100%)
- **Station:** Location of the presenting part in relation to the midpelvis or ischial spines, measured in centimeters above and below, using a scale from −5 to + 5 or −3 to + 3
  - Station 0 = engaged
  - Station + 2 = 2 cm below the level of the ischial spines
  - + 5 = crowning
- **Fetal presentation:** part of the fetus that presents to the inlet
- **Position:** relationship of the point of reference (occiput sacrum, acromion) on the fetal presenting part to the mother's pelvis
  - Left occiput anterior (LOA): most common position

Labor Progression Cont'd.

- **Lie:** relationship of the long axis (spine) of the fetus to the long axis (spine) of the mother
  - Longitudinal: up and down
  - Transverse: perpendicular
  - Oblique: slanted
- **Attitude:** relationship of fetal parts to one another
  - Flexion: desired attitude, so that smallest diameter of the fetal head is presented
  - Extension can cause dystocia

Prolapsed Cord: knee chest position to relieve compression.

Nursing and Collaborative Management

Assessment
- Baseline maternal vital signs including pain
- Medication history
- Physical assessment
  - Nutrient and fluid intake: hydration and bladder status, need for catheterization, intravenous (IV) therapy
  - Bowel elimination
  - Ambulation and positioning: upright, sitting, squatting (best position)
  - Labs and diagnostic tests
- Emotional and cultural responses

Nursing and Collaborative Management Cont'd.

Labor Assessment

•Onset of labor and progression

•Vaginal exam (assess dilation, effacement, station, position, and fetal presentation; do not perform in the presence of bleeding, which could indicate placenta previa or abruption.)

•Status of membranes

•Show

•FHR pattern

•Complications: infection, pregnancy-induced hypertension (PIH) or gestational hypertension, bleeding, prolapsed cord, fetal distress

Nursing and Collaborative Management, Cont'd.

Assessment of contractions (uterine activity pattern)

• *Duration:* amount of time a contraction lasts, from the beginning to the end

• *Frequency:* the time from the beginning of one contraction to the beginning of the next contraction

•*Intensity:* internal monitoring from 30 mm Hg (mild) to 70 mm Hg (strong)

•*Resting tone/time:* tension of uterine muscle between contractions and time between contractions

Fetal Heart Rate

Characteristics of the fetal heart rate (FHR)

•**Normal range**: 110 to 160 beats/min

•**Tachycardia**: >160 beats/min

•**Bradycardia**: <110 beats/min

•**Variability**: change in the heart rate from beat to beat (short term) and cyclic changes over time (long term), in 3 to 5 cycles per minute; moderate long-term variability is reassuring

Changes in Fetal Heart Rate

Accelerations: FHR increases with movement; reassuring

Decelerations:

- Early decelerations (reassuring) often occur during second stage and indicate head compression.
- Late decelerations (nonreassuring): even if not very "deep," indicate placental insufficiency or hypoxia.
- Variable decelerations (nonreassuring): may or may not be associated with contractions, indicate compression of umbilical cord.
- The deceleration pattern indicates the insult to the fetus; the variability indicates how well the fetus is tolerating the insult.

Fetal Monitoring

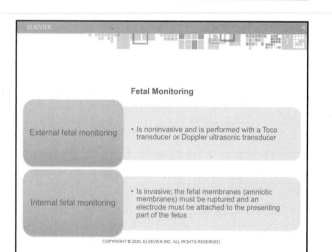

External fetal monitoring	• Is noninvasive and is performed with a Toco transducer or Doppler ultrasonic transducer
Internal fetal monitoring	• Is invasive; the fetal membranes (amniotic membranes) must be ruptured and an electrode must be attached to the presenting part of the fetus

Question

A woman who is in labor becomes nauseated, starts hiccupping, and tells her partner to leave her alone. The partner asks the nurse what he did to make this happen. Which response should the nurse provide?

A. "In active labor, it is quite common for women to react this way. It's nothing you did."

B. "I don't know what you did, but stop, because she is quite sensitive right now."

(C) "I'll come and examine her. This reaction is common during the transition phase of labor."

D. "Early labor can be very frustrating. I'm sure she doesn't mean to take it out on you."

Nursing and Collaborative Care During Labor

Assessment

- Cultural factors: influence response to labor and coping
- Emotional response: support and coping
- Pain and discomfort: medications and nonpharmacological measures
- Response to medications: epidural and oxytocin
- Maternal vital signs
- Fetal heart rate pattern
- Uterine activity
- Fetal position—Leopold's maneuvers and vaginal exam

Assessment of Labor Progression dilatation, effacement, descent

- Status of the membranes: prevent and detect infection
- Nutrient and fluid intake: hydration and bladder status, need for catherization, IV therapy
- Bowel elimination
- Labs and diagnostic tests
- Signs of complications: infection, pregnancy induced hypertension (PIH), bleeding, prolapsed cord, fetal distress
- Ambulation and positioning; upright, sitting, squatting

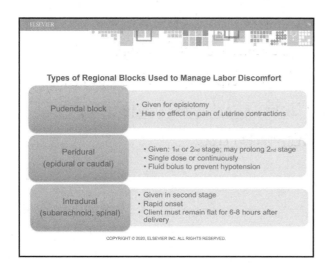

Types of Regional Blocks Used to Manage Labor Discomfort

Pudendal block	• Given for episiotomy • Has no effect on pain of uterine contractions
Peridural (epidural or caudal)	• Given: 1st or 2nd stage; may prolong 2nd stage • Single dose or continuously • Fluid bolus to prevent hypotension
Intradural (subarachnoid, spinal)	• Given in second stage • Rapid onset • Client must remain flat for 6-8 hours after delivery

---

Handwritten notes:

Timing of epidural: lateral part of 1st stage or early 2nd.
· hypotension is common after: give fluids. Epidural ↑ risk of urine retention post-partum.

Drugs Used During Labor

Narcotics: inhibit contractions if given before well-established labor; can cause respiratory depression if given too close to birth; antidote is naloxone.

- Fentanyl
- Morphine sulfate
- Hydromorphone

Mixed agonist/antagonists: use these drugs with caution in substance abusers, as they could cause withdrawal in narcotics users.

- Butorphanol tartrate
- Nalbuphine

Postpartum Maternal Assessment Memory Tool: BUBBLE HA

Breasts
- Assess consistency (soft, firm, filling, engorged), nipples (intact, sore, flat, everted or inverted), masses

Uterus Fundal Involution
- Immediately after delivery: fundus is several centimeters below umbilicus
- Within 12 hours: fundus rises to umbilicus
- Descends 1 cm (fingerbreadth) a day for 9 to 10 days; then fundus is below symphysis pubis
- Should be in midline and firm

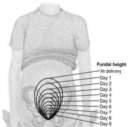

Fundal height
- At delivery
- Day 1
- Day 2
- Day 3
- Day 4
- Day 5
- Day 6
- Day 7
- Day 8
- Day 9

Postpartum Maternal Physical Assessment: BUBBLE HA

Bladder
- Measure output; assess for distention or retention

Bowel
- Assess for distention, passing flatus, and bowel sounds

Lochia
- Endometrial sloughing from rubra (red); serosa (pink); alba (white)
- Assess color, odor, volume

Leg Assessment
- Assess for signs of thrombosis

Episiotomy
- Assess episiotomy or laceration repair for intactness, hematoma, edema, bruising, redness, and drainage

Hemorrhoids
- Treat with: Sitz bath; Tucks; ointments

Attachment
- Assess maternal-infant interaction for bonding behaviors

Rubra: 3-4 /days
Serosa: 3-4 / days
Alba: up to a few weeks.
· Unrelieved pain: developing hematoma.

Teaching Points

Primary focus is on signs of physical and emotional symptoms of potential problems for mother and infant.

- Change peri pads as needed and with voiding/defecation
- Wipe perineum front to back
- Good handwashing technique
- Ice packs, sitz baths, peri bottle lavage, and topical anesthetic spray and pads
- Breastfeeding instructions ✗
- Balanced diet and adequate fluid intake
- Rest/nap when baby sleeps
- Contraceptive use

postpartum blues: 2 wks (norm)

Reinforce Teaching Points

RhoGAM

- Given to Rh-negative women with possible exposure to Rh-positive blood
- Should have negative indirect Coombs' test
- Given IM within 72 hours after delivery
- Checked by two nurses (blood product)

Rubella Vaccine

- Given subcutaneously to nonimmune client before discharge from hospital
- May breastfeed
- Do not give if client or family member is immunocompromised.
- Avoid pregnancy for 2 to 3 months (reinforce contraception)

Question

A client who is 72 hours post cesarean section is preparing to go home. She complains to the nurse that she can't get the baby's diaper on right. Which action should the nurse take?

A. Demonstrate how to diaper the baby correctly

B. Observe the client diapering the baby while offering praise and hints

C. Call the social worker for long-term follow-up

D. Reassure the client that she knows how to take care of her baby

Complications of Childbearing

Chronic Hypertension

Hypertension and/or proteinuria in pregnant woman:
- Chronic hypertension before 20 weeks of gestation
- Persistent after 12 weeks postpartum

Superimposed Preeclampsia or Eclampsia

Development of preeclampsia or eclampsia in woman with chronic hypertension before 20 weeks of gestation

---

Question

A client at 33 weeks' gestation who has been diagnosed with pregnancy-induced hypertension (PIH) is admitted to the labor and delivery area. The client expresses concern for the health of her baby. Which response should the nurse make?

A. "You have the best doctor on the staff, so don't worry about a thing."

B. "Your anxiety is contributing to your condition and may be the reason for your admission."

C. "This is a minor problem that is easily controlled, and everything will be all right."

D. "As I assess you and your baby, I will explain the plan for your care and answer your questions."

Preeclampsia/Eclampsia

Preeclampsia Symptoms		
	Mild	Severe
BP	BP rise to 30 mm Hg systolic and 15 mm Hg diastolic over previous baseline, or 140/90 or greater	BP of 160/110 mm Hg, when either diastolic reaches 160 mm Hg or systolic reaches 110 mm Hg, or both occur simultaneously. Can be confirmed within a short interval.
Proteinuria	≥1+ (≥0.3 g in a 24-hour specimen)	2+ to 3+ (2 g in a 24-hour specimen)
Edema	Eyes, face, fingers	Generalized edema
DTR	May be normal	3+ or greater and clonus
CNS Symptoms	Headache, irritability	Severe headache, visual disturbances
Other	Weight gain >2lbs/week; oliguria <100 mL/4h; epigastric pain, ↑creatinine, thrombocytopenia, marked SGOT elevation	

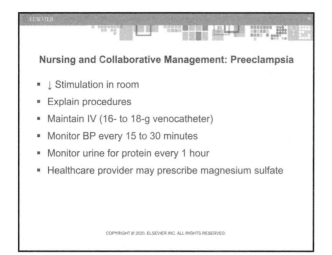

Nursing and Collaborative Management: Preeclampsia

- ↓ Stimulation in room
- Explain procedures
- Maintain IV (16- to 18-g venocatheter)
- Monitor BP every 15 to 30 minutes
- Monitor urine for protein every 1 hour
- Healthcare provider may prescribe magnesium sulfate

Nursing and Collaborative Management: Eclampsia (Seizures)

- Stay with client
- Turn client to side
- Notify HCP if client starts having seizures
- Do not attempt to force objects into client's mouth
- Remember that seizures can occur postpartum
- Administer oxygen and have suction available

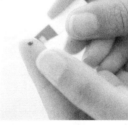

Gestational Diabetes

Screening

- 1-hour glucose screen between 24 and 26 weeks
- Goal: strict blood glucose control
- Generally, Glyburide or insulin is used during pregnancy.
- Insulin does not cross the placenta, and Glyburide only minimally crosses it

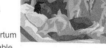

· Most oral hypoglyumics cross the plaunta.

Question

A client with gestational diabetes asks the nurse to explain the reason her baby is at risk for macrosomia. Which explanation should the nurse offer?

A. The placenta receives decreased maternal blood flow during pregnancy because of vascular constriction.

(B) The fetus secretes insulin in response to maternal hyperglycemia, causing weight gain and growth.

C. Infants of diabetic mothers are postmature, which allows the fetus extra time to grow.

D. Rapid fetal growth contributes to congenital anomalies, which are more common in infants of diabetic mothers.

Preterm Labor (PTL)

Signs and Symptoms

- More than five contractions in an hour
- Feels like menstrual cramps
- Low, dull backache
- Pelvic pressure
- Increase/change in vaginal discharge
- Leaking or gush of amniotic fluid

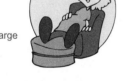

PTL: Tocolytics and Their Administration

MEDICATIONS	SIDE EFFECTS	ADVERSE EFFECTS	NURSING INTERVENTIONS	ANTIDOTE
Terbutaline	Nervousness	Tachycardia	Maternal pulse >130 BPM; arrhythmias, chest pain	Propranolol
	Tremulousness	Chest pain	BP <90/60 mm Hg	Beta-blocker
	Headache	Pulmonary edema	Pulmonary edema	
	N/V, diarrhea	Low K⁺	FHR 1 >180 BPM	
	Epigastric pain	Hyperglycemia	Hyperglycemia in women treated with steroids	
			I & O, daily weight	
Magnesium sulfate	CNS depression	↓ Urine output	Hold if R <12 , urine output <100 mL/4 h, absent DTRs	Calcium gluconate
	↓ Respirations and DTRs	Pulmonary edema	Monitor magnesium levels.	

PTL: Other Drugs Used to Decrease Contractions

- Indomethacin, naproxen
- Fenoprofen
- Nifedipine
- Nicardipine

Drug to Enhance Fetal Lung Maturity
- Betamethasone
- Used if fetus is <35 weeks' gestation

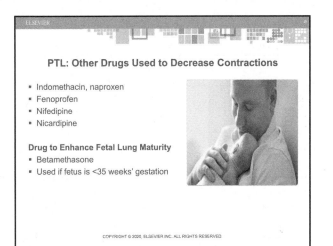

Spontaneous Abortion

Assessment
- Vaginal bleeding at week 20 or less of gestation
- Uterine cramping, backache, and pelvic pressure
- May have symptoms of shock
- Assess client's and family members' emotional status, needs, and provide support

Nursing and Collaborative Management
- Monitor VS, LOC, and amount of bleeding
- Prepare client to receive IV fluids and/or blood
- If client is Rh negative, administer RhoGAM

Question

A client at 15 weeks' gestation is admitted for an inevitable abortion. Thirty minutes after returning from surgery, her vital signs are stable. Which intervention has the highest priority?

A. Ask the client if she would like to talk about losing her baby.

B. Place cold cabbage leaves on the client's breasts to decrease breast engorgement.

C. Send a referral to the grief counselor for at-home follow-up.

D. Confirm the client's Rh and Coombs' status and administer RhoGAM if indicated.

Handwritten note: Concern: hypovolemia — hemodynamic stability

Incompetent Cervix

Recurrent premature dilation of the cervix; is defined as passive and painless dilation of the cervix during the second trimester

- **Conservative management**
  - ✓ Bed rest
  - ✓ Hydration
  - ✓ Tocolysis (inhibition of uterine contractions)
- **Cervical cerclage may be performed**
  - ✓ Postoperative nursing care: monitor uterine activity, bleeding, and rupture of membranes, and signs of infection.
- **Administer tocolytics**
  - Discharge teaching: teach to report signs of labor, bleeding, and infection; decrease activity to 1 week and pelvic rest.

Ectopic Pregnancy

Assessment
- Missed period, but early signs of pregnancy absent
- Positive pregnancy test

Rupture
- Sharp, unilateral pelvic pain
- Vaginal bleeding
- Referred shoulder pain
- Syncope can lead to shock

Nursing and Collaborative Management
- Monitor hemodynamic status
- Prepare client for surgery and administration of IV fluids, including blood

★ hypovolemia

Abruptio Placentae and Placenta Previa

	Abruptio Placentae	Placenta Previa
Bleeding	Concealed or overt	Bright red vaginal (usually in third trimester)
Uterine Tone	Tense without relaxation to rigid and board like	Soft
Pain	Persistently painful	Painless
Fetal Heart Rate	Usually abnormal (complete abruption = absent FHR)	Usually normal unless bleeding is severe and mother becomes hypovolemic

- Abruptio placenta: painful —
  ↑ mortality
- Placenta Previa: ∅ pain
  ∅ abdominal, vaginal asx —
  can complicate things.

DIC and Dystocia

Disseminated Intravascular Coagulation
Risk factors for DIC in pregnancy:
- Fetal demise
- Infection/sepsis
- Pregnancy-induced hypertension (preeclampsia)
- Abruptio placentae

Dystocia
A difficult birth resulting from problems involving the "5 Ps" (**P**owers, **P**assage, **P**assenger, **P**syche, and/or **P**osition). Examples include a lack of progress in cervical dilation, delay in fetal descent, or change in the characteristics of uterine contraction.

Postpartum Complications

Hemorrhage
- Assess fundal location and consistency
- Assess vaginal bleeding; saturating one pad/hour indicates hemorrhage.
- Monitor for signs of shock
- Assess for bladder distention; can prevent involution and lead to hemorrhage

Venous Thromboembolism
- Related to venous stasis and hypercoagulability
- Can result in superficial venous thrombosis, deep vein thrombosis, or pulmonary embolism
- Assess legs for pain, tenderness, swelling (Homan's sign not reliable)
- Treated with bed rest, anticoagulants, leg elevation, and analgesia

Postpartum Infections

Infection
- Perineal infections
- Endometritis
- Parametritis
- Peritonitis
- Mastitis
- Cystitis
- Deep vein thrombosis
- Pyelonephritis
- HIV, hepatitis, other sexually transmitted infections

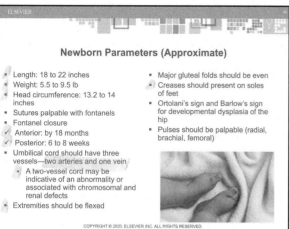

Newborn Parameters (Approximate)

- Length: 18 to 22 inches
- Weight: 5.5 to 9.5 lb
- Head circumference: 13.2 to 14 inches
- Sutures palpable with fontanels
- Fontanel closure
  - Anterior: by 18 months
  - Posterior: 6 to 8 weeks
- Umbilical cord should have three vessels—two arteries and one vein
  - A two-vessel cord may be indicative of an abnormality or associated with chromosomal and renal defects
- Extremities should be flexed
- Major gluteal folds should be even
- Creases should present on soles of feet
- Ortolani's sign and Barlow's sign for developmental dysplasia of the hip
- Pulses should be palpable (radial, brachial, femoral)

BP norm: 70's / 50's

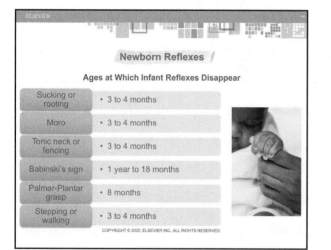

Newborn Reflexes

Ages at Which Infant Reflexes Disappear

Sucking or rooting	3 to 4 months
Moro	3 to 4 months
Tonic neck or fencing	3 to 4 months
Babinski's sign	1 year to 18 months
Palmar-Plantar grasp	8 months
Stepping or walking	3 to 4 months

jaundice begins: head →
chest → extremities.
50 kcal / day / 6 mo

Newborn Nursing and Collaborative Management

- Keep newborn warm ✗
- Suction airway as needed
- Observe for respiratory distress
- Normal or physiological jaundice appears after the first 24 hours in full-term newborns ✗
- Pathological jaundice occurs before this time and may indicate early ★ hemolysis of red blood cells
- Assess the hemoglobin and hematocrit (H&H) and blood glucose levels
- Weigh daily
- Monitor intake and output; weigh diapers if necessary (1 g = 1 mL of urine)
- Monitor temperature
- Observe for any cracks in skin
- Administer eye medication within 1 hour after birth
- Provide cord care
- Provide circumcision care; teach client how to care for circumcision site
- Supine position ("Back to sleep") to prevent SIDs
- Observe for normal stool and passage of meconium
- Test the newborn's reflexes

Question

Which nursing action has the highest priority for an infant immediately after birth?

A. Place the infant's head in the "sniff" position and give oxygen via face mask.

B. Perform a bedside glucose test and feed the infant glucose water as needed.

C. Assess the heart rate and perform chest compressions if rate is <60 beats/min.

D. Dry the infant and place him or her under a radiant warmer or skin to skin with the mother.

Major Newborn Complications: Hypoglycemia

- Assess for risk factors in maternal history (infant of diabetic mother) and environmental factors (cold stress)
- In general, blood glucose levels <40 mg/dL are considered abnormal and warrant investigation and intervention
- Infant is fed formula or breastfed as soon as the repeat (usually) sample is obtained to prevent a further drop in blood glucose
- Administer IV glucose infusions per HCP prescription for infants with symptomatic hypoglycemia or those too ill to be safely fed orally
- Reduce adverse environmental factors (e.g., excessive handling and cold stress)

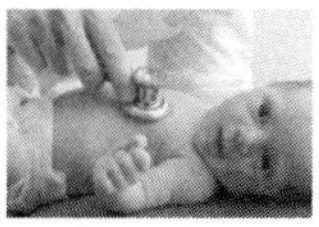

Major Newborn Complications

Respiratory Distress Syndrome
- Caused by inability to produce surfactant
- Resulting in hypoxia and acidosis

Meconium Aspiration Syndrome
- Fetal distress increases intestinal peristalsis.
- Releases meconium into the amniotic fluid

Retinopathy of Prematurity
- Damage to retinal vessels caused by prolonged use of oxygen (>30 days)
- Infants receiving oxygen should be examined by ophthalmologist

---

Handwritten notes:

T - ABC
↳ temperature

Major Newborn Complications: Hyperbilirubinemia

- ↑ Serum levels >12 mg/dL
- Crucial to prevent of kernicterus, which results in permanent neurological damage
- Jaundice starts at the head, spreads to the chest, abdomen, arms, legs, hands, and feet

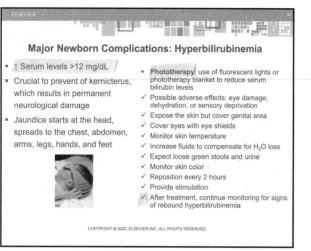

- **Phototherapy**, use of fluorescent lights or phototherapy blanket to reduce serum bilirubin levels
- ✓ Possible adverse effects: eye damage, dehydration, or sensory deprivation
- ✓ Expose the skin but cover genital area
- ✓ Cover eyes with eye shields
- ✓ Monitor skin temperature
- ✓ Increase fluids to compensate for H_2O loss
- ✓ Expect loose green stools and urine
- ✓ Monitor skin color
- ✓ Reposition every 2 hours
- ✓ Provide stimulation
- ✓ After treatment, continue monitoring for signs of rebound hyperbilirubinemia

---

Major Newborn Complications: Erythroblastosis Fetalis

- Results from Rh- mother exposed to Rh+ blood and develops antibodies that are passed to the fetus, destroying fetal red blood cells
- Characterized by hemolytic anemia or hyperbilirubinemia
- Exchange of fetal and maternal blood occurs at birth
- Administer $Rh_o(D)$ immune globulin to Rh- mother to prevent development of maternal antibodies
- Treatment of newborn includes phototherapy and exchange transfusions

---

Major Newborn Complications

Sepsis
- Presence of bacteria in the blood
- Prevention—antibiotics in labor for group B *Streptococcus* (GBS) positive test
- Assess for maternal, intrapartum, and neonatal risk factors
- Early signs are nonspecific and include lethargy, poor feeding, poor weight gain, and irritability

TORCH Infections
- Infections that are caused by one of the following:
  - **T**oxoplasmosis
  - **O**ther infections (e.g., gonorrhea, syphilis, varicella, hepatitis B, HIV, or human parvovirus B19)
  - **R**ubella
  - **C**ytomegalovirus
  - **H**erpes simplex virus

Green urine/stool: NORMAL S/E of phototherapy.

newborn ↑ aspiration risk when
eating due to "sniffling" when
eating.

Major Newborn Complications

Maternal Substance Abuse
- Effects on fetus vary according to substance
- Narcotics cause passive addiction: neonatal abstinence syndrome
- Cocaine is classified as a narcotic but not an opioid; it causes vasoconstriction, preterm birth, poor growth, neurological problems

Fetal Alcohol Syndrome
- Caused by maternal alcohol use during pregnancy
- Associated with neurological problems, IQ deficit, and attention-deficit/hyperactivity disorder
- Craniofacial features include microcephaly, small eyes or short palpebral fissures, a thin upper lip, a flat midface, and an indistinct philtrum.
- Treatment of drug-exposed newborns focuses on reduction of external stimuli, supportive treatment of symptoms, and sedation.

Major Newborn Complications

Maternal HIV

PCR testing <18mo

- Monitor antibodies closely throughout pregnancy
- Testing and treatment in pregnancy greatly reduce risk of transmission to fetus

Maternal Diabetes
- Infant born to mother with type 1 or type 2 diabetes or gestational diabetes
- Newborn may have hypoglycemia, hypocalcemia, hypomagnesemia, polycythemia, hyperbilirubinemia, cardiomyopathy, respiratory distress syndrome (RDS), birth trauma, and congenital anomalies

Jittery newborn: can be glucose or
Ca^+ problem.

Question

A pregnant client tells the nurse that she drinks only one glass of wine a day. Which information should the nurse provide the client about the effects of drinking alcohol during pregnancy?

A. Alcohol causes vasoconstriction and decreases placental perfusion.

B. Alcohol decreases the lecithin:sphingomyelin (L:S) ratio, contributing to lung immaturity.

C. Alcohol causes vasodilation and increased fluid overload for the fetus.

(D.) Alcohol during pregnancy places the fetus at risk for fetal alcohol spectrum disorders.

L:S ratio : 2:1 target for
surfactant development.

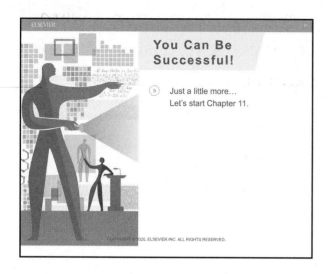

Mental Health Nursing

Mental Health Nursing

Nurse-Client Relationship

The goal of the nurse-client relationship is to facilitate quality client-centered care by using verbal and nonverbal communication to build trust, provide comfort, and encourage change.

Privacy and Confidentiality

A client's reasonable expectation is that information revealed to the nurse will not be disclosed to others. However, the nurse must explain to the client that information relevant to the individual's treatment plan must be shared with the other members of the treatment team, especially if the client has thoughts of harm to self or others.

Mental Health Nursing

Therapeutic Communication
- Both *verbal* and *nonverbal* expression
- Goal-directed
- Appropriate, efficient, flexible, and based on the client's ability to provide feedback

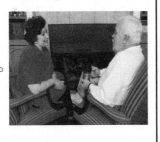

Therapeutic Communication

Principles
- Establish trust
- Demonstrate a nonjudgmental attitude
- Offer self; be empathetic, not sympathetic
- Use active listening
- Accept and support client's feelings
- Clarify and validate client's statements
- Use matter-of-fact approach

Examples of Therapeutic Communication
- **Silence**: sit quietly and wait
- **Active listening**: give full attention to the client
- **Open-ended questioning**: promotes sharing
- **Empathizing**: demonstrates warmth and acknowledgment of feelings
- **Restating**: repeat what the client says to show understanding and to review what was said

Mental Health Definitions

Mental Health
- A lifelong process
- Successful adjustment to changing environments (internal and external)

Mental Illness
- Defined by clinically significant behavior as a result of the client's distress or disability
- An inability to respond to the environment because of mental or medical conditions that affect the client's thinking, ability to relate to others, mood, feeling, and daily functioning (e.g., impaired thinking, poor impulse control, or altered behavior)
- In many clients, it is a temporary loss, while in others, it may be a lifelong series of intermittent exacerbations of illness

Cognitive-behavioral therapy for coping mechanisms.

Question

An adult client is admitted to the inpatient mental health unit with a diagnosis of severe depression. As the client begins to recover, the client develops rapport with the nurse. After being discharged from the hospital, the client and the nurse happen to meet in the coffee shop. The client asks the nurse if they can schedule future meetings at the coffee shop. Which response by the nurse is most therapeutic?

- A. "I'll contact the nurse supervisor about this plan."
- B. "Let's not plan to meet; however, we may inadvertently see each other here."
- C. "It's not appropriate for me to discuss therapy with you when I'm off duty."
- D. "A social relationship with a former client is not appropriate."

Question

A female client who is a 5-year breast cancer survivor received confirmation that she has a recurrence of breast cancer. She informs her family that the biopsy was negative. What action should the nurse take?

- A. Tell the client's family to consult the healthcare provider.
- B. Ask the client to restate what the healthcare provider told her.
- C. Encourage the client to inform her family about the results.
- D. Suggest the client talk to the nurse about her fears.

Coping and Defense Mechanisms

- Primarily unconscious efforts to decrease anxiety
- Can be constructive or destructive
- Coping is related to problem solving
- Defense is related to protecting oneself
  - Denial
  - Displacement
  - Identification

Therapeutic Treatment Modalities

Milieu Therapy: the physical, social, and therapeutic environment in which the client is receiving treatment

Collaborative Care: the hallmark of treatment in mental health. The team includes nurses, psychiatrists, social workers, mental health technicians, drug/alcohol therapists, etc.

Interpersonal Psychotherapy: uses a therapeutic relationship to modify the client's feelings, attitudes, and behaviors

Behavior Therapy: includes many formats that are used to assist the client in changing behavior

Cognitive Therapy: directive, time-limited approach

Crisis Intervention: directed at resolution of the immediate crisis and to returning the individual to the precrisis level of functioning

Electroconvulsive Therapy (ECT): infrequently used treatment that uses controlled electrically induced seizures to treat severely depressed individuals who fail to respond to antidepressant medications and therapy

ECT S/E: memory loss, nausea, seizure.

Question

During the initial phase, a group member, who has a master's degree, states, "My educational background makes it easier for me to help the other group members." Which action should the nurse take to assure effective group functioning?

- A. Reiterating the purpose of the support group sessions
- B. Asking the group to identify various stressful problems
- C. Obtaining ideas from the members about strategies for stressful situations
- D. Terminating the meeting and evaluate the situation

Group Therapy

- Involves a therapist and five to eight members
- Provides feedback and support for the individual goals of each member
- Group therapy models:
  - Stress management
  - Self-care
  - Medication education
  - Dual diagnosis
  - Cognitive behavioral therapy (CBT)

- Interpersonal group therapy
- Self-help or support groups
- Family therapy
  - The member with the presenting symptoms indicates the presence of problems in the entire family
  - A change in one member will bring about changes in other members

Therapeutic Factors of Groups

- **Instillation of hope and optimism** about group treatment
- **Universality:** Members realize they are not alone with their problems, feelings, or thoughts
- **Imparting of information:** Members receive formal teaching by the leader or advice from peers
- **Altruism:** Members feel a reward from giving support to others

- **Recapitulation:** Members repeat patterns of behavior in the group that they learned in their families; feedback from the leader and peers provides opportunities to learn about their behavior
- **Development of socializing techniques:** Members learn new social skills based on feedback from others
- **Imitative behavior:** Members copy behavior from the leaders or peers and can adopt healthier habits

Therapeutic Factors in Groups

- **Interpersonal learning:** Members gain insight into themselves based on feedback from others; occurs later in group after establishing trust.
- **Group cohesiveness:** In a mature group, members accept positive feedback and constructive criticism.

- **Catharsis:** Intense feelings, as judged by the member, are shared.
- **Existential resolution:** Members learn to accept painful aspects of life (i.e., loneliness, death) that affect everyone.

Stages of Group Development

- **Initial Stage:** superficial communication
- **Working Stage:** real work is done by group; nurse and client orient to parameters of a therapeutic relationship
- **Termination Stage:** provides opportunity to learn to deal with letting go

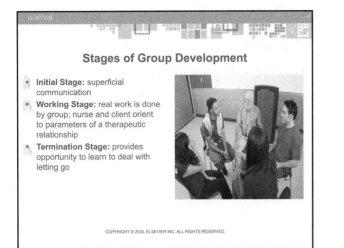

Question

The nurse and the unlicensed assistive personnel (UAP) take a group of mental health clients to a baseball game. During the game, a client reports shortness of breath and dizziness. Which intervention should the nurse implement first?

- A. Have the UAP escort the client back to the unit.
- B. Request that the client describes current feelings.
- C. Accompany the client to a quiet area.
- D. Ask the client if anything untoward occurred.

Anxiety

Mild or moderate anxiety is a normal subjective experience that includes feeling of apprehension, uneasiness, uncertainty, or dread.

Types of Anxiety

- Mild: tension of everyday life
- Moderate: immediate concerns
- Severe: feeling that something bad is about to happen
- Panic: terror and a sense of impending doom

Immediately intervene during panic anxiety. Common w/ GAD

Anxiety Disorders

Generalized Anxiety Disorder

- An unrealistic or persistent anxiety about everyday worries
- Panic disorders produce a sudden feeling of intense apprehension.

Phobias

- Irrational fear of an object, activity, or situation
- Client may or may not recognize fear as unreasonable
- Associated with panic-level anxiety
- Defense mechanisms include repression and displacement (i.e., agoraphobia)

Nursing and Collaborative Management

- Reduce environmental stimuli
- Provide a calm, quiet environment
- Administer antianxiety medications
- Administer SSRIs and tricyclic antidepressants

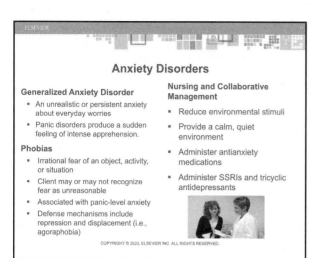

Question

The nurse is planning to teach client strategies for coping with anxiety. The nurse finds the client engaged in compulsive handwashing. What action should the nurse take next?

A. While the client is handwashing, introduce alternatives to handwashing.
B. Ask the client to immediately stop handwashing; then begin teaching.
C. Allow client to complete handwashing; then begin teaching.
D. Ask client to describe events that precipitated the handwashing.

Antianxiety (Anxiolytic) Medication

- Benzodiazepines:
  - Recommended for only short-term use because these drugs are addictive and may depress the central nervous system
  - Have anxiety-reducing (anxiolytic), sedative-hypnotic, muscle-relaxing, and anticonvulsant actions

- Flumazenil (Anexate; Romazicon): a benzodiazepine antagonist administered intravenously that reverses benzodiazepine intoxication in 5 minutes

---

Handwritten notes

- Benzo's: Short-term anxiety "-pams"
- Anti-depressents

- Flumazenil Ø work immediately. Takes 5-10 min

Somatic Symptom Disorder (DSM-5)

Persistent worry or statements regarding physical illness without physical findings

- **Types of somatic symptom disorders:**
  - Illness anxiety disorder or somatic disorder is a preoccupation with complaints about chronic symptoms that cause significant distress.
  - Factitious disorders are self-imposed fabricated symptoms (aka Munchhausen syndrome).
  - Factitious disorder by proxy occurs when symptoms are imposed on another, e.g., parent induces illness in child (aka, Munchhausen by proxy).
- **Treatment:** cognitive behavioral therapy — *ongoing*

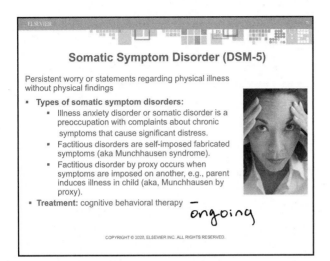

Crisis Intervention

Crisis

Results from experiencing a significant traumatic event or situation that cannot be remedied by the use of previous coping strategies.

Risk Factors

- Multiple comorbidities and losses
- Unexpected life changes
- Limited coping skills
- Chronic pain or disability
- Poor social support
- Concurrent psychiatric disorders, substance abuse, or disability
- Limited access to healthcare service

Goal

Return client to precrisis level of functioning

Nursing and Collaborative Management

- Assess for suicidal or homicidal thoughts or plans
- Help client feel safe and less anxious
- Listen carefully
- Be directive (e.g., nurse may arrange for shelter or contact a social worker)
- Mobilize social support
- Involve client in identifying realistic, acceptable interventions
- Regular follow-up is not usually part of crisis intervention

Trauma Stressor Related Disorders

Acute Stress

- Abnormal response to an extreme abnormal event (witnessing a horrific car accident or war-zone blast)

Acute Stress Disorder

- Occurs within a month after an individual experiences or sees an event involving death, severe injury, or physical violation to the individual or others

Posttraumatic Stress Disorder

- Reexperience of traumatic event involving (or real threat of) death, serious injury, or physical violation
- May experience recurrent and intrusive dreams or flashbacks
- Associated with four clusters:
  - Avoidance of reminders
  - Symptoms of numbing
  - Alterations in behavior including self-destructive (suicide), aggression, and irritability
  - Persistent negative mood and alterations in in cognition

Handwritten notes:

Safety Concerns: 1) projecting illness onto someone else
2.) prescriptions from multiple MD. Risk of OD (polypharmacy)

• Is there homicidal or suicidal ideation?

Nursing and Collaborative Management

- Implement suicidal and homicidal precautions as needed.

- Consistently provide nonthreatening environment.

- Actively listen to client's description of events to identify the most troubling aspects.

- Assist the client in identifying past successes to promote client's ability to regain control.

Dissociative Disorders

These disorders are rarely encountered and are an unconscious defense mechanism that protects the person against overwhelming anxiety

- **Dissociative amnesia:** a sudden temporary inability to recall important personal events following a traumatic event
- **Dissociative amnesia with fugue:** one or more episodes of an inability to recall important information, usually of a traumatic nature
- **Dissociative identity disorder:** two or more distinct identities, at least two of which recurrently take control
- **Depersonalization or derealization disorder:** persistent or recurrent episodes of feelings of detachment from oneself that occurs in response to acute stress

Personality Disorders

Obsessive-Compulsive Disorder
- *Obsessive*
  - Persistently intrusive thoughts
- *Compulsive*
  - Repetitive behaviors designed to divert unacceptable thoughts and reduce anxiety (e.g., compulsive handwashing)

Antisocial Personality Disorder
- Aggressive toward others without remorse
- Is manipulative, self-centered, and impulsive

Borderline Personality Disorder
- Highly changeable and intense affect
- Poor impulse control, engages in self-damaging behavior (e.g., sexual and/or suicidal)
- Pits perceived good person (nurse, friend, family member) against perceived bad person; switches which person is good

Associated behaviors
- Inflexible maladaptive behavior patterns
- In touch with reality
- Lacks insight into behavior
- Poor impulse control
- Forms of acting out include:
  - ✓ Yelling and swearing
  - ✓ Cutting own skin
  - ✓ Manipulating others
  - ✓ Abusing substances
  - ✓ Engaging in promiscuous sexual behaviors
  - ✓ Attempting suicide

Handwritten notes:
- Consistant boundaries, consequences, + accountability.

Question

A client diagnosed with borderline personality disorder returns after a weekend pass with lacerations to both wrists. The client complains about how the nurse is performing the dressing change. The nurse's response should be presented in which manner?

A. Disinterested
B. Concerned
C. Matter-of-fact
D. Empathetic

Eating Disorders

Compulsive Overeating
- Binge-like overeating without purging
- Lack of control over food consumption

Anorexia Nervosa
- Onset is often associated with a stressful event
- Death can occur from starvation, suicide, cardiomyopathies, or electrolyte imbalance
- The client experiences an altered body image

Bulimia Nervosa
- Binge-purge syndrome in which eating binges are followed by purging behaviors

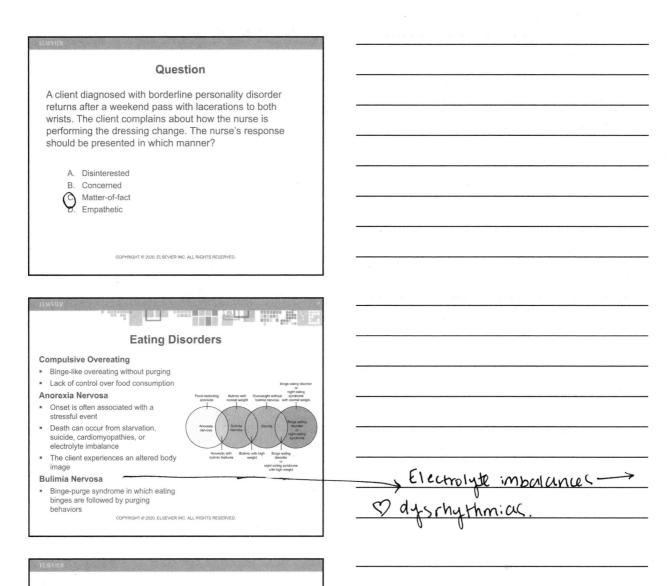

→ Electrolyte imbalances →
♡ dysrhythmias.

Question

A client diagnosed with a history of bulimia is admitted to the mental health unit. What intervention is most important for the nurse to include in the initial treatment plan?

A. Observe the client after meals for purging.
B. Assess daily weight and vital signs.
C. Monitor serum potassium and calcium.
D. Provide a structured environment at mealtime.

Question

The mental health RN is assigned to five clients. Which clients should have priority assessments? (Place in order of priority.)

A. A newly admitted client diagnosed with major depression whose assessment is incomplete

B. A client diagnosed with schizophrenia who is having auditory hallucinations of an infant crying

C. A client who has a 5-year history of daily consumption of two six-packs of beer

D. A client diagnosed with bulimia who is having difficulty attending group

E. A client who has been taking benzodiazepines off and on daily for the last 2 years

Depressive Disorders

Major Depressive Disorder

- Dysthymia (persistent depressive disorder)
- Premenstrual dysphoric disorder
- Substance/medication-induced depressive disorder
- Depressive disorder used by another medical condition

Depression

- Characterized by feelings of hopelessness, low self-esteem, self-blame
- Some 25% of those diagnosed with depression have suicidal ideation.
- Clients respond well to behavioral therapy, cognitive behavioral therapy, and interpersonal psychotherapy.
- Antidepressant medication therapy
  - Tricyclic antidepressants (e.g., TCAs; sometimes referred to as cyclic antidepressants)
  - SSRIs and SNRIs
  - Atypical antidepressants

Suicide

- A suicide threat is a warning, direct or indirect, verbal or nonverbal, that a person is planning to take his or her own life.
- Assessment includes whether the person has made a specific plan and whether the means to carry out the plan are available.
- **NEVER** leave a suicidal client alone.
- Protect the client from inflicting self-harm, be vigilant, supervise medication administration, implement strategies to ↑ self-esteem and social support.

Suicide Precautions

- ✓ Ongoing observations and monitoring of the client
- ✓ Provide protective environment
- ✓ Search for weapons or potential weapons.
- Be aware of major warning signs of an impending attempt
  - Client begins to give away possessions
  - Makes a will or funeral arrangements
  - Client suddenly becomes "better" or "happy"

Bipolar Disorder

Bipolar Disorder

Characterized by mood swings involving depression, euphoria, grandiosity, and an inflated sense of self-worth

Medications (Mood Stabilizers)

- Lithium carbonate: medication of choice; can be toxic and requires regular monitoring of serum lithium levels
- Toxic level is >1.2 mEq/L

Other Medications

- Divalproex (Valproate)
- Olanzapine (Zyprexa)
- Carbamazepine (Tegretol)

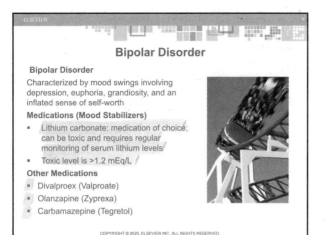

Monoamine Oxidase Inhibitors (MAOIs)

Use caution when administering MAOIs.

- Inhibit the enzyme monoamine oxidase, which is present in the brain, blood platelets, liver, spleen, and kidneys.
- Administered to clients with depression who have not responded to other antidepressant therapies, including ECT
- There must be a 2-week wash-out period between using MAOIs and SSRIs or SNRIs (in either direction, i.e., from MAOI to SSRIs, or vice versa); otherwise, the mixture can trigger a hypertensive crisis.

- Concurrent use with the following may cause **hypertensive crisis**: tyramine-containing foods (red wine, aged cheese, smoked meats, pickles, sauerkraut, etc.), amphetamines, antidepressants, dopamine, opioids epinephrine, guanethidine, levodopa, methyldopa, nasal decongestants, norepinephrine, reserpine, or vasoconstrictors.

- Concurrent use with opioid analgesics may cause hyper- or hypotension, coma, or seizures.

SNRIs, SSRIs, and TCAs

- Serotonin and norepinephrine reuptake inhibitors (SNRIs) block reabsorption of serotonin and norepinephrine
- Selective serotonin reuptake inhibitors (SSRIs)
  - ✓ Inhibit serotonin uptake
- Tricyclic antidepressants (TCAs)
  - ✓ Block the reuptake of norepinephrine (and serotonin) at the presynaptic neuron
  - ✓ May take several weeks to produce the desired effect (2 to 4 weeks after the first dose)
  - ✓ NOTE: Trazodone can cause priapism. Priapism affects the penis and in rare instances, the clitoris.

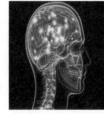

· Educate taking lithium even if feeling better. Keep Na⁺ levels steady.

Antidepressant Medications

Antidepressant Medications	Action	Side Effects/Considerations
SSRI Citalopram (Celexa) Escitalopram (Lexapro) Fluvoxamine (Luvox) Fluoxetine (Prozac) Paroxetine (Paxil) Sertraline (Zoloft)	Inhibit serotonin reuptake	Drowsiness, dizziness, headache, insomnia, depressed appetite
Tricyclic antidepressants (TCAs) Amitriptyline Clomipramine (Anafranil) Desipramine (Norpramin) Imipramine (Tofranil) Nortriptyline Protriptyline (Vivactil) Trimipramine (Surmontil)	Block reuptake of NE at pre-synaptic neurons	May take 2 to 4 weeks to produce effect Tachycardia, dizziness, insomnia, drowsiness, fluid retention

HIGH-ALERT Antidepressant Use

Serotonin Syndrome
- Hyperthermia, rigidity, cognitive impairments, and autonomic symptoms
- Potentially fatal and may occur at any time during therapy with SSRIs or SNRIs (serotonin norepinephrine reuptake inhibitor) combined with MAOIs
- Treatment is symptomatic with propranolol, cooling blankets, chlorpromazine for hyperthermia, diazepam for muscle rigidity or rigors

Antidepressant apathy: Some clients lose interest in life and the events around them (related to SSRIs)

Antidepressant withdrawal syndrome: Abrupt cessation of antidepressants engenders withdrawal symptoms

Antidepressant loss of effectiveness: Sometimes medications are no longer effective

Antidepressant-induced suicide: Especially 18- to 24-year-olds in the early stages of treatment

HIGH-ALERT Antidepressant Use

Lithium toxicity is *potentially fatal.*

- Hyperthermia as high as 108° F (42.2° C), cognitive impairments, and autonomic symptoms
- Muscular rigidity
- Altered mental status
- Irregular pulse
- Cardiac dysrhythmias
- Diaphoresis

Nursing and Collaborative Management
- ***Immediately*** discontinue lithium
- Client may need to transfer to a critical care unit

- Up to 6 wks for symptom relief.
- Begin w/ SSRI's.
- Tricyclic: more ♡ problems.

Question

Today's lab report of the lithium level is 1.3 mEq/mL for a client diagnosed with bipolar disorder. Which is the first action the nurse should take?

A. Withhold the dose until after breakfast
B. Give the client the prescribed dose
C. Obtain a prescription to increase the dose
D. Withhold the dose and notify the healthcare provider

Schizophrenia Spectrum and Other Psychotic Disorders

A group of mental disorders characterized by psychotic features

Key Symptoms of Schizophrenia
- Delusions (thoughts or beliefs)
- Hallucinations
- Disorganized speech
- Negative symptoms

Positive Symptoms
- Hallucinations and delusions

Perceptual Distortions
- Difficulty understanding or using information

Illusions
- Brief experiences of mi sperception of reality that usually occur with delirium, DTs, or drug induced

Hallucinations
- Perceptions without a basis in reality
- Includes five senses (smell, touch, etc.)

Delusions
- False beliefs

Safety is the first priority!

Antipsychotic Medications

Traditional Medications
- Chlorpromazine
- Haloperidol (Haldol)

Purpose: Treat psychotic behavior

Side Effects
- Extrapyramidal (EPS)
- Akathisia
- Acute dystonia
- Pseudoparkinsonism
- Anticholinergic

Nursing Assessment
- Screen for EPS using Abnormal Involuntary Movement Scale (AIMS).
- Encourage fluid, gum, and hard candy, and increase fiber intake

Long-Acting Medications
- Clozapine (Clozaril)
- Risperdal (risperidone) Long-Acting Injection

Side Effects
- Blood dyscrasias and neuroleptic malignant syndrome (very high fever)

Nursing and Collaborative Management
- Teach patient to change positions slowly to prevent dizziness, and report urinary retention.
- Stress importance of maintaining medication therapy.

Atypical Medications
- Aripiprazole (Abilify)

Purpose: treat all positive and negative symptoms

Side effects: multiple side effects depending on medication

Nursing assessment: tolerance to effects, NMS

*Harsh S/E
Haldol: Parkinsonian
long-acting / atypical:
neuroleptic malignant syndrome
STOP the antipsychotic

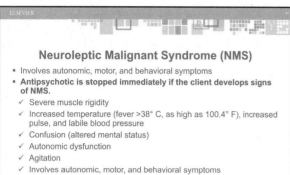

Neuroleptic Malignant Syndrome (NMS)

- Involves autonomic, motor, and behavioral symptoms
- **Antipsychotic is stopped immediately if the client develops signs of NMS.**
  - ✓ Severe muscle rigidity
  - ✓ Increased temperature (fever >38° C, as high as 100.4° F), increased pulse, and labile blood pressure
  - ✓ Confusion (altered mental status)
  - ✓ Autonomic dysfunction
  - ✓ Agitation
  - ✓ Involves autonomic, motor, and behavioral symptoms
- Associated medications
  - ✓ Haloperidol, Fluphenazine, Trifluperazine, Thioridazine, Loxapine, Clozaril, Risperidone, Olanzapine, Ziprasidone, Reserpine, Droperidol, Lithium, Levodopa, Desipramine, Amantadine

---

Nursing and Collaborative Management

- Assess for risk of violence to self or others and take appropriate precautions
- Provide quiet, soothing environment
- Establish routine and boundaries
- Provide stable, nonthreatening, brief, social interactions
- If client is acting frightened or scared, increase your distance of physical space surrounding the client and approach client calmly
- Encourage reality-based interests

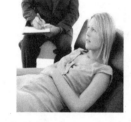

Substance Abuse Disorders

- **Substance dependence:** a pattern of repeated use of a substance
- **Substance tolerance:** a need for more of the substance to reach the desired effect
- **Substance abuse:** recurrent use of a substance
- **Substance withdrawal:** symptoms occur when blood levels of a substance decline

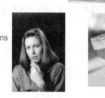

✶ Routine!

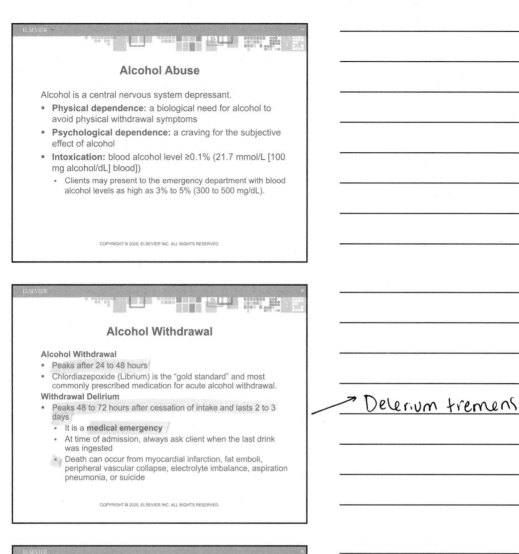

Alcohol Abuse

Alcohol is a central nervous system depressant.

- **Physical dependence:** a biological need for alcohol to avoid physical withdrawal symptoms
- **Psychological dependence:** a craving for the subjective effect of alcohol
- **Intoxication:** blood alcohol level ≥0.1% (21.7 mmol/L [100 mg alcohol/dL] blood])
  - Clients may present to the emergency department with blood alcohol levels as high as 3% to 5% (300 to 500 mg/dL).

Alcohol Withdrawal

Alcohol Withdrawal
- Peaks after 24 to 48 hours
- Chlordiazepoxide (Librium) is the "gold standard" and most commonly prescribed medication for acute alcohol withdrawal.

Withdrawal Delirium
- Peaks 48 to 72 hours after cessation of intake and lasts 2 to 3 days
  - It is a **medical emergency**
  - At time of admission, always ask client when the last drink was ingested
  - Death can occur from myocardial infarction, fat emboli, peripheral vascular collapse, electrolyte imbalance, aspiration pneumonia, or suicide

→ Delerium tremens

Disulfiram (Antabuse) Therapy

- Alcohol deterrent
  - Instruct the client who is on disulfiram therapy to avoid the use of substances that contain alcohol, such as:
    - Cough medicines
    - Mouthwashes
    - Aftershave lotions
- Other medications used to assist with alcohol cravings:
  - Acamprosate calcium
  - Naltrexone

Question

A client with a history of alcohol abuse is admitted to the medical unit for gastrointestinal bleeding and pancreatitis. The admission data include BP 156/96 mm Hg, pulse 92 beats/min, and temperature 37.3° C (99.2° F). Which intervention is most important for the nurse to implement?

A. Provide a quiet, low-stimulus environment

B. Initiate seizure precautions

C. Administer as-needed (PRN) lorazepam (Ativan) as prescribed

D. Determine the time and quantity of the client's last alcohol intake

---

Autism Spectrum Disorder

- **Etiology:** no known cause
- **Clinical Description**
  - ✓ Hyperactivity
  - ✓ Short attention span
  - ✓ Impulsivity
  - ✓ Aggressivity
  - ✓ Self-injurious behavior
  - ✓ Temper tantrums
  - ✓ Repetitive mannerisms
  - ✓ Preoccupation with objects
  - ✓ Absence of spoken language
  - ✓ "Islands of genius"

Prognosis
- No known cure
- Language skills and intellectual level are strongest factors related to prognosis
- Only a small percentage of individuals with the disorder go on to live and work independently as adults

---

Attention-Deficit/Hyperactivity Disorder

Etiology: No known cause, but there is a strong correlation between genetic factors and ADHD

Clinical Description

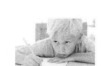

- Fidgeting in a seat
- Getting up when expected to be seated
- Excessive running when it is dangerous or inappropriate
- Loud and disruptive play during quiet activities
- Forgets and misses appointments
- Fails to meet deadlines
- Loses the train of conversation
- Changes topics inappropriately
- Does not follow rules of games

Attention-Deficit/Hyperactivity Disorder

Treatment with CNS stimulants may be required to reduce hyperactive behavior and lengthen attention span.

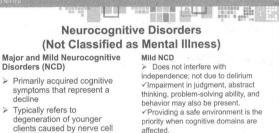

Prognosis
- Continues into adolescence in the majority of children
- Many adults with ADHD in childhood report a decrease of hyperactivity but a continuation of difficulty concentrating or attending to complex projects

Clients with attention-deficit/hyperactivity disorder may require CNS stimulants to reduce hyperactive behavior and lengthen attention span.

Neurocognitive Disorders
(Not Classified as Mental Illness)

Major and Mild Neurocognitive Disorders (NCD)

- ➤ Primarily acquired cognitive symptoms that represent a decline
- ➤ Typically refers to degeneration of younger clients caused by nerve cell deterioration (e.g., traumatic brain injury, HIV)

Symptoms

- ✓ Significant cognitive decline
- ✓ Interference with independent functioning
- ✓ Not caused by other mental disorder

Mild NCD
- ➤ Does not interfere with independence; not due to delirium
- ✓ Impairment in judgment, abstract thinking, problem-solving ability, and behavior may also be present.
- ✓ Providing a safe environment is the priority when cognitive domains are affected.

Cognitive Domains
- ✓ Learning and memory
- ✓ Language
- ✓ Perceptual-motor
- ✓ Social cognition
- ✓ Executive function
- ✓ Complex attention

Neurocognitive Disorders

- ➤ Dementia is NOT classified by DSM-5 as mental illness.
- ➤ DSM-5 refers to major and mild neurocognitive disorders (NCD) terminology (sometimes referred to as dementia).

Dementia: Progressive deterioration in intellectual functioning secondary to structural or functional changes

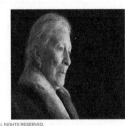

- Long-term and short-term memory loss
- Impairment in judgment, abstract thinking, problem-solving ability, and behavior
- Caused by nerve cell deterioration
- Providing a safe environment is the priority

#Safety Priority

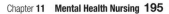

Alzheimer's Disease

- Irreversible form of senile dementia caused by nerve cell deterioration
- Priority is client safety.
- Maintain comfort, toilet as necessary; keep dry
- Reduce environmental stimulation during late afternoon and evening
- Maintain daily routine
- Provide environmental cues; turn on lights before dusk; provide night-light
- Provide soothing music
- Provide reassurance and companionship, especially during difficult evening period

Neurocognitive Disorders: Medications

- Donepezil (Aricept)
- Galantamine (Razadyne)
- Memantine (Namenda)
- Rivastigmine (Exelon)
- Tacrine

- Aricept: Slows progression of ~~dementia.~~ Alzheimer's.

Question

A 68-year-old client who is diagnosed with Alzheimer's disease is admitted to the nursing home by the nurse. The client does not recognize spouse or children and forgets how to eat and dress. What is the nurse's priority intervention for the newly admitted client?

A. Establish a daily routine and schedule

B. Encourage involvement in structured activities

C. Discuss strategies to coordinate care

D. Stress the importance of self-nurturing

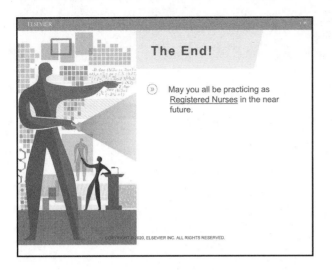

The End!

» May you all be practicing as
Registered Nurses in the near
future.

Type Cancer	Risk Factors/ Symptoms	Diagnostics/Classifications	Treatment Options	Nursing Considerations
Leukemia (can be acute or chronic)	The cause, although unknown, is attributed to genetic origin, viral infection, previous treatment with or exposure to radiation, or chemotherapeutic agents.	Blood results and bone marrow examination are the primary methods of diagnosing and classifying the type of leukemia. **Common findings** Decreased platelet count and hemoglobin WBC count to be low, elevated, or excessively elevated Bone marrow biopsy shows immature leukocytes. Chest radiographic examination may show mediastinal lymph node and lung involvement and bone changes. Lymph node biopsy reveals excessive blasts (immature cells). Further studies such as lumbar puncture and CT scan can be performed to determine the presence of leukemic cells outside of the blood and bone marrow. **Classifications of leukemia** Chronic lymphocytic leukemia (CLL): CLL affects lymphoid cells (cells that become lymphocytes, often B cells) and usually grows slowly. It accounts for more than 15,000 new cases of leukemia each year. Most often, people diagnosed with the disease are over age 55. It almost never affects children. **Chronic myeloid leukemia (CML):** CML affects myeloid cells (cells that become any type of blood cell other than lymphocytes) and usually grows slowly at first. It accounts for nearly 5000 new cases of leukemia each year. It mainly affects adults. **Acute lymphocytic (lymphoblastic) leukemia (ALL):** ALL affects lymphoid cells and grows quickly. It accounts for more than 5000 new cases of leukemia each year. ALL is the most common type of leukemia in young children. It also affects adults. **Acute myeloid leukemia (AML):** AML affects myeloid cells and grows quickly. It accounts for more than 13,000 new cases of leukemia each year. It occurs in both adults and children.	**Acute** Treatment is aimed at eradicating the leukemia with multidrug chemotherapy and/ or bone marrow transplant, and/or hematopoietic stem cell transplantation (HSCT). **Chronic** Treatment is dependent on the kind of cells involved. Medications commonly used include chlorambucil (Leukeran), hydroxyurea, corticosteroids, and cyclophosphamide. Lymph nodes are often irradiated, and blood transfusion may be given if anemia is severe. Although medications are not curative in chronic leukemia, they help to prolong life.	Prevent infections Monitor for bleeding Pain management Encourage a diet high in calories, protein, and vitamins, as well as soft, bland food Monitor for side effects and toxicities of treatment agents Support coping mechanisms

Type Cancer	Risk Factors/ Symptoms	Diagnostics/Classifications	Treatment Options	Nursing Considerations
Multiple Myeloma (malignant neoplastic disease of the bone marrow)		Radiographic skeletal studies, bone marrow biopsy, and blood and urine specimens—**monoclonal antibody (M protein)** Common findings include pancytopenia, hypercalcemia, hyperuricemia, and elevated creatinine. **Bence Jones protein** is found in the urine and can result in renal failure.	Treatment is symptom management since multiple myeloma is not curable. Small-dose radiation and chemotherapy may be used; proteasome inhibitors (newer treatment option).	Pain management Prevent infection. Prevent bone injury. Encourage weight-bearing exercises. Encourage 3–4 liters/day. Monitor for side effects of chemotherapy.
Hodgkin's Lymphoma	Occurs twice as often in men as women. Peak targets two primary age ranges: Early adulthood (15–30 years) and around 50 years. No major risk factors but seen commonly in people with mononucleosis, acquired or congenital immunodeficiency syndromes, those taking immunosuppressive drugs after organ transplantation, those who have been exposed to occupational toxins, or have a genetic predisposition. The presence of HIV increases the incidence of Hodgkin's lymphoma. Symptoms include painless enlargement of the cervical, axillary or inguinal lymph nodes, anorexia, weight loss, fever, night sweats, malaise, and extreme pruritus.	Lymph node biopsy—**Reed Sternberg cell** CXR MRI or PET scan Anemia Low iron, albumin Elevated calcium, alkaline phosphatase **Clinical Staging System for Hodgkin's Disease** **Stage I** • Abnormal single lymph nodes • Regional or single extranodal site **Stage II** • Two or more abnormal lymph nodes on the same side of the diaphragm • Localized involvement of extranodal site and one or more lymph node regions on the same side of the diaphragm **Stage III** • Abnormal lymph node regions on both sides of the diaphragm • May be accompanied by spleen involvement • Now subdivided into lymphatic involvement of the upper abdomen in the spleen (splenic, celiac, and portal nodes) (stage III1) and the lower abdominal nodes in the periaortic, mesenteric, and iliac regions (stage III2) **Stage IV** Diffuse and disseminated involvement of one or more extralymphatic tissues and/or organs—with or without lymph node involvement; the extranodal site is identified as H, hepatic; L, lung; P, pleural; M, marrow; D, dermal; and O, osseous	The stage guides the treatment. Combination chemotherapy for early stage; chemotherapy and radiation for later stages. Bone marrow or peripheral stem cell transplantation (SCT) also considered for later stages.	Skin care Temperature management Monitor for side effects of treatment, therapies. Emotional support

Type Cancer	Risk Factors/ Symptoms	Diagnostics/Classifications	Treatment Options	Nursing Considerations
Non-Hodgkin's Lymphoma (NHL): group of malignant neoplasms of primarily B- or T-cell origin, affecting people of all ages. Common names for different types of lymphoma include Burkitt's lymphoma, diffuse large B-cell lymphoma, lymphoblastic lymphoma, and follicular lymphoma.	No known cause but previous infection with human T-cell leukemia/ lymphoma virus and the Epstein-Barr virus have been found to be linked to the disease. More common in men over 60 years of age. Symptoms include painless, enlarged lymph nodes and fever, weight loss, night sweats, anemia, pruritus, fatigue. Because of the progression of the disease, at the time of diagnosis other symptoms are very possible based on spread (i.e., enlarged liver, pleural effusions, or bone fractures).	Biopsies of lymph nodes, liver, and bone marrow; bone scan, PET scan, MRI CBC Most common staging for NHL—low grade (indolent), intermediate grade (aggressive), and high grade (very aggressive).	Chemotherapy and radiation Monoclonal antibody-rituximab (Rituxan); Ibritumomab (Zevalin) Tumor necrosis factor Interferon therapy	Prevent infections. Monitor for side effects related to treatment therapies.
Brain tumors (can be benign or malignant)	Genetic predisposition Environmental Headache (worse in the morning), dizziness, new-onset seizures, change in LOC, personality, or cognition	CT scan (most often used) MRI, PET scan, EEG Stereotactic biopsy,	Surgery (craniotomy/ craniectomy using a surgical navigation system) Chemotherapy/ radiation	Ongoing assessment for changes from baseline or new symptoms Monitor for signs of increased ICP. CSF leakage (meningitis) Infection

Type Cancer	Risk Factors/ Symptoms	Diagnostics/Classifications	Treatment Options	Nursing Considerations
Breast	The cause is unknown. Primary risk factors: gender (female), age (greater than 50 years), race (North American or Northern European descent), family history (two or more first-degree relatives with the disease, and a first-degree relative with bilateral premenopausal breast cancer), genetics (BRCA1 and BRCA2) Breast tumors are usually small, solitary, irregularly shaped, firm, nontender, and nonmobile. There may be a change in skin color, feelings of tenderness, puckering or dimpling of tissue (peau d'orange— skin with the appearance and texture of an orange peel), nipple discharge, retraction of the nipple, and axillary tenderness.	Self-breast exam (>90% of tumors are discovered by the client) Clinical breast exam (a 1 cm tumor is discoverable to physical exam) Mammogram (can detect a 0.5 cm tumor) Biopsy (sentinel lymph node mapping may be used prior to standard lymph node biopsy) MRI, PET scan Estrogen and progesterone receptor status	Treatment based on the type and stage of cancer Radiation, chemotherapy, and surgery alone or in combination may be used. Hormone therapy Tamoxifen Toremifene (Fareston) Letrozole (Femara) Bisphosphonates- pamidronate sodium (Aredia) Raloxifene (Evista) megestrol (Megace) Monoclonal antibody trastuzumab (Herceptin) (used in metastatic breast cancer for clients that express the cancer cell antigen HER2) Bone marrow and stem cell transplantation	Clients scheduled for mastectomy: Emotional support (anticipatory grieving; body image acceptance) Wound management Monitor for infection. Hemodynamic stability Post-mastectomy arm exercises Educate about avoiding any procedures involving the arm on the affected side—blood pressure readings, injections, IV infusion of fluids, or the drawing of blood, which may cause edema or infection. Monitoring for side effects of treatment therapies

Type Cancer	Risk Factors/ Symptoms	Diagnostics/Classifications	Treatment Options	Nursing Considerations
Cervical	Risk factors linked to sexual behavior (multiple partners and sexually active in teenage years), STIs with several strains of HPV, and smoking. Vague to no symptoms in the early stages (spotting between menses); vaginal bleeding increasing in amount and with an odor and pain in the back and thighs in the later stages	Pap test; physical examination; colposcopy and cervical biopsy; and additional diagnostic studies, such as a computed tomography (CT) scan, chest radiographic evaluation, IV pyelogram, cystoscopy, sigmoidoscopy, or liver function studies to determine the extent of invasion	Preventative strategies- vaccinations Gardasil; Cervarix Carcinoma in situ— electrocautery, laser, conization, and hysterectomy. Early carcinoma— hysterectomy or intracavitary radiation Late carcinoma— radical hysterectomy with pelvic lymph node dissection; radiation (either external or brachytherapy), chemotherapy (cisplatin-based)	Education about early detection and treatment Pain management Nutritional status Vaginal drainage (amount, color, odor)
Colorectal	Cause unknown Risk factors include age (>50), other disease processes (polyps, ulcerative colitis, and diverticulosis), family history, diet, smoking, excessive intake of alcohol, obesity, and diabetes	Fecal occult blood testing Colonoscopy CT scan Decreased hemoglobin	Radiation Chemotherapy Surgery (bowel resection)	Based on treatment options For client scheduled for surgery with colostomy: Pre-op teaching includes management of bag-barrier device; post-op expectations- change in body image, fears/ concerns Stoma should always be pink and moist; mild edema may be expected 1–2 weeks post-op.
Prostate	Onset insidious with the nodule on the posterior portion of the prostate; later symptoms of urinary obstruction and hematuria	Digital rectal examination PSA Biopsy The Gleason grading system Score of 2–4 indicates a slow-progressing tumor. Score of 5–7 indicates a more aggressive tumor.	Radiation (external or brachytherapy) Hormone therapy Luteinizing hormone–releasing hormone (LHRH) agonist—leuprolide (Lupron) and goserelin (Zoladex); LHRH antagonist- Degarelix (Firmagon) Radical prostatectomy	Based on treatment options

From Cooper, K., & Gosnell, K. (2015). *Adult health nursing* (7th ed.). St. Louis, MO: Elsevier/Mosby.

Test	Adult	Child	Infant/Newborn	Elder	Nursing Implications
			Hematological		
Hgb (hemoglobin): g/dL or mmol/L (SI units) **Possible critical values <5.0 or >20 g/dL**	Male: 14–18 g/dL or 8.7–11.2 mmol/L Female: 12–16 g/dL or 7.4–9.9 mmol/L Pregnant: >11 g/dL	1–6 years: 9.5–14 g/dL 6–18 years: 10–15.5 g/dL	Newborn: 14–24 g/dL 0–2 weeks: 12–20 g/dL 2–6 months: 10–17 g/dL 6 months–1 year: 9.5–14 g/dL	Values slightly decreased	High-altitude living increases values. Drug therapy can alter values. Slight Hgb decreases normally occur during pregnancy.
Hct (hematocrit): volume fraction (SI units) or % **Possible critical values <15% or >60%**	Male: 0.42–0.52 volume fraction or 42%–52% Female: 0.37–0.47 volume fraction or 37%–47% Pregnant: >33%	1–6 years: 30–40 6–18 years: 32–44	Newborn: 44–64 2–8 weeks: 39–59 2–6 months: 35–50 6 months–1 years: 29–43	Values slightly decreased	Prolonged tourniquet application can cause stasis and alter values. Abnormalities in RBC size may alter Hct values.
RBC (red blood cell) count: RBC × 10^{12}/L (SI units)	Male: 4.7–6.1 Female: 4.2–5.4	1–6 years: 4–5.5 6–18 years: 4–5.5	Newborn: 4.8–7.1 2–8 weeks: 4–6 2–6 months: 3.5–5.5 6 months–years: 3.5–5.2	Same as adult	Never draw a specimen from an arm with an infusing IV. Exercise and high altitudes can cause an increase in values. Values are usually lower during pregnancy. Drug therapy can alter values.
WBC (white blood cell) count: WBC × 10^9/L (SI units) **Possible critical values <2500 or >30,000 mm^3**	Both genders: 5000–10,000 mm^3 or 5–10 × 109/L	≤2 years: 6200–17,000 mm^3 ≥2 years: 5000–10,000 mm^3 or 5–10 × 109/L	Newborn: 9,000–30,000/mm^3	Same as adult	Anesthetics, stress, exercise, and seizures can cause increased values. Certain types of drugs can increase or decrease WBC levels. The final month of pregnancy and labor may cause increased WBC levels.

Test	Adult	Child	Infant/Newborn	Elder	Nursing Implications
Platelet count: × 10^9/L (mm³) **Possible critical values <50,000 or >1 million/mm³**	Both genders: 150,000–400,000 mm³ or 150–400 × 109/L (SI units)	150,000–400,000 mm³	Premature infant: 100,000–300,000 mm³ Newborn: 150,000–300,000 mm³ Infant: 200,000–475,000 mm³	Same as adult	Living at high altitudes, exercising strenuously, or taking oral contraceptives may increase values. Decreased values may be caused by hemorrhage, DIC, reduced production of platelets, infections, use of prosthetic heart valves, and drugs (e.g., chemotherapy, H2 blockers, INH, levofloxacin, streptomycin, sulfonamides, thiazide diuretics).

HESI Hint: The laboratory values that are most important to know for the NCLEX–RN exam are Hgb, Hct, WBCs, Na⁺, K⁺, BUN, blood glucose, ABGs (arterial blood gases), bilirubin for newborns, and therapeutic range for PT and PTT.

Test	Adult	Child	Infant/Newborn	Elder	Nursing Implications
SED rate, ESR (erythrocyte sedimentation rate): mm/hr	Male: up to 15 mm/hr Female: up to 20 mm/hr	Up to 10 mm/hr	Newborn: 0–2 mm/hr	Same as adult	Pregnancy (second and third trimester) can cause elevations in ESR.
PT (prothrombin time): sec	Both genders: 11–12.5	Same as adult	Same as adult	Same as adult	PT is monitored to help regulate warfarin (Coumadin) dosages. Therapeutic range: 1.5–2 times normal or control
PTT (partial thromboplastin time): sec (see APTT, below)	Both genders: 60–70	Same as adult	Same as adult	Same as adult	PTT is monitored to help regulate heparin dosages. Therapeutic range: 1.5–2.5 times normal or control
INR (international normalized ratio)	Both genders: 0.8–1.1	Same as adult	Same as adult	Same as adult	Ideal INR value must be individualized. Typical values for certain clients: Clients with atrial fibrillation and deep vein thrombosis, between 2.0 and 3.0 Clients with mechanical heart valves, between 3.0 and 4.0
APTT (activated partial thromboplastin time): sec	Both genders: 30–40 Pregnancy may prolong APTT	Same as adult	Same as adult	Same as adult	APTT is used to help partially regulate heparin dosages. Therapeutic range: 1.5–2.5 times normal or control

Test	Adult	Child	Infant/Newborn	Elder	Nursing Implications
Blood Chemistry					
Alkaline phosphatase: units/L	Both genders: 30–120	<2 years: 85–235 2–8 years: 65–210 9–15 years: 60–300 16–21 years: 30–200		Slightly higher than adult	Hemolysis of specimen can cause falsely elevated values.
Albumin: g/dL or g/L (SI units)	Both genders: 3.5–5 g/dL or 35–50 g/L	4.5–9 g/dL	Premature infant: 3–4.2 g/dL Newborn: 3.5–5.4 g/dL Infant: 4.4–5.4 g/dL	Same as adult	No special preparation is needed.
Bilirubin total: mg/dL or μmol/L (SI units)	Total: 0.3–1.0 mg/dL or 5.1–17 μmol/L Indirect: 0.2–0.8 mg/dL or 3.4–12.0 μmol/L Direct: 0.1–0.3 mg/dL or 1.7–5.1 μmol/L	Same as adult	Newborn: Total bilirubin: 1.0–12.0 mg/dL or 17.1–205 μmol/L	Same as adult	Prevent hemolysis of blood during venipuncture. Do not shake tube; this can cause inaccurate values. Protect blood sample from bright light.
Hematological					
Calcium: mmol/L (mg/dL)	Both genders: 2.25–2.75 (9–10.5)	2.2–2.7 (8.8–10.8)	<10 days: 1.9–2.60 (7.6–10.4) Cord: 2.25–2.88 (9–11.5) 10 days–2 years: 2.3–2.65 (9–10.6)	Values tend to decrease.	No special preparation is needed. Use of thiazide diuretics can cause increased calcium values.
Chloride: mmol/L (SI units) or mEq/L	Both genders: 98–106	90–110	Newborn: 96–106 Premature infant: 95–110	Same as adult	Do not collect from an arm with an infusing IV solution.
Cholesterol: mmol/L (SI units) or mg/dL	Both genders: <5.2 mmol/L or <200 mg/dL	120–200 mg/dL	Infant: 70–175 mg/dL Newborn: 53–135 mg/dL	Same as adult	Do not collect from an arm with an infusing IV solution.
CPK (creatine phosphokinase): units/L	Male: 55–170 Female: 30–135	Same as adult	Newborn: 65–580	Same as adult	Values are higher after exercise. Early pregnancy may cause decreased levels.
Creatinine: μmol/L (SI units) or mg/dL	Female: 0.5–1.1 mg/dL or 44–97 μmol/L Male: 0.6–1.2 mg/dL or 53–106 μmol/L	Adolescent: 0.5–1.0 mg/dL Child: 0.3–0.7 mg/dL	Infant: 0.2–0.4 mg/dL Newborn: 0.3–1.2 mg/dL	Decrease in muscle mass may cause decreased values.	NPO for 8 hr before testing is preferred but not required. BUN-to-creatinine ratio of 20:1 indicates adequate kidney functioning.
Glucose: mmol/L (SI units) or mg/dL	Both genders: 74–106 mg/dL or 4.1–5.9 mmol/L	Child <2 years: 60–100 mg/dL or 3.3–5.5 mmol/L Child >2 years to adult: Fasting (no caloric intake for at least 8 hr): 70–110 mg/dL or <6.1 mmol/L Nonfasting: ≤200 mg/dL (<11.1 mmol/L)	Cord: 45–96 mg/dL or 2.5–5.3 mmol/L Premature infant: 20–60 mg/dL or 1.1–3.3 mmol/L Neonate: 30–60 mg/dL or 1.7–3.3 mmol/L Infant: 40–90 mg/dL or 2.2–5.0 mmol/L	60–90 years: 82–115 mg/dL or 4.6–6.4 mmol/L >90 years: 75–121 mg/dL or 4.2–6.7 mmol/L	Client is kept NPO, except for water, for 8 hours before testing. Stress, infection, and caffeine can cause increased values

Test	Adult	Child	Infant/Newborn	Elder	Nursing Implications
HCO₃–: mmol/L (mEq/L)	Both genders: 21–28	21–28	Newborn/infant: 16–24	Same as adult	None
Iron: μmol/L (SI units) or mcg/dL	Male: 80–180 mcg/dL or 14–32 μmol/L Female: 60–160 mcg/dL or 11–29 μmol/L	50–120 mcg/dL	100–250 mcg/dL	Same as adult	NPO for 12 hours before test.
TIBC (total iron binding capacity): μmol/L (SI units) or mcg/dL	Both genders: 250–460 mcg/dL or 45–82 μmol/L	Same as adult	Same as adult	Same as adult	None
LDH (lactic dehydrogenase): units/L	Both genders: 100–190	60–170	Newborn: 160–450 Infant: 100–250	Same as adult	Do not give IM injections for 8–12 hours before test. Hemolysis of blood causes a false–positive result.
Potassium: mmol/L (SI units) or mEq/L	Both genders: 3.5–5	3.4–4.7	Newborn: 3.9–5.9 Infant: 4.1–5.3	Same as adult	Hemolysis of specimen can result in falsely elevated values. Exercise of the forearm with tourniquet in place may cause an increased potassium level.
Protein total: g/L (SI units) or g/dL	Both genders: 6.4–8.3 g/dL or 64–83 g/L	6.2–8 g/dL	Premature infant: 4.2–7.6 g/dL Newborn: 4.6–7.4 g/dL Infant: 6–6.7 g/dL	Same as adult	NPO for 8 hours before test is preferred but not required.
AST/SGOT (aspartate aminotransferase): units/L	0–35 Female slightly lower than adult male	3–6 years: 15–50 6–12 years: 10–50 12–18 years: 10–40	0–5 days: 35–140 <3 years: 15–60	Slightly higher than adult	Exercise may cause an increased value. If possible, avoid giving any IM injection because increased enzyme levels may result.
ALT/SGPT (alanine aminotransferase): units/L	Both genders: 4–36	Similar to adult	Values may be 2 × as high as adults	Slightly higher than adult	Previous IM injections may cause elevated levels.
Sodium: mEq/L	Both genders: 136–145	136–145	Newborn: 134–144 Infant: 134–150	Same as adult	Recent trauma, surgery, or shock may cause increased levels.
Triglycerides: mmol/L (SI units) or mg/dL	Male: 40–160 mg/dL or 0.45–1.81 mmol/L Female: 35–135 mg/dL or 0.40–1.52 mmol/L	Male 6–11: 31–108 mg/dL 12–15: 36–138 mg/dL 16–19: 40–163 mg/dL Female 6–11: 35–114 mg/dL 12–15: 41–138 mg/dL 16–19: 40–128 mg/dL	Male 0–5: 30–86 mg/dL Female 0–5: 32–99 mg/dL	Same as adult	Client is kept NPO for 12 hours before test. No alcohol for 24 hours before test

Test	Adult	Child	Infant/Newborn	Elder	Nursing Implications
BUN (blood urea nitrogen): mmol/L (SI units) or mg/dL	Both genders: 10–20 mg/dL or 3.6–7.1 mmol/L	5–18 mg/dL	Infant: 5–18 mg/dL Newborn: 3–12 mg/dL Cord: 21–40 mg/dL	Slightly higher	None
Arterial Blood Chemistry					
pH	Both genders: 7.35–7.45	Child >2 years: same as adult	Newborn: 7.32–7.49 2 months–2 years: 7.34–7.46	Same as adult	Specimen must be heparinized. Specimen must be iced for transport. All air bubbles must be expelled from sample. Direct pressure to puncture site must be maintained.
PCO$_2$: mm Hg	Both genders: 35–45	Same as adult	<2 years: 26–41	Same as adult	See above.
PO$_2$: mm Hg	Both genders: 80–100	Same as adult	Newborn/Infant: 60–70	Same as adult	See above.
HCO$_3$–: mmol/L (mEq/L)	Both genders: 21–28	Same as adult	Newborn/Infant: 16–24	Same as adult	See above.
O$_2$ saturation: %	Both genders: 95–100	Same as adult	Newborn: 40–90	95	See above.

BUN, Blood urea nitrogen; *DIC,* disseminated intravascular coagulation; *DVT,* deep vein thrombosis; *IM,* intramuscular; *INH,* isoniazid; *NPO,* nothing by mouth; *PCO$_2$,* carbon dioxide partial pressure; *PO$_2$,* oxygen partial pressure; *HCO$_3$–,* bicarbonate.

From Pagana, KD, Pagana, TJ, Pagana TN. (2019). *Mosby's Diagnostic and Laboratory Test Reference.* 14th ed. St. Louis, MO: Elsevier.

Appendix C
Comparison of Three Types of Hepatitis

Characteristics	Hepatitis A (Infectious Hepatitis)	Hepatitis B (Serum Hepatitis)	Hepatitis C
Source of Infection	■ Contaminated food ■ Contaminated water or shellfish	■ Contaminated blood products ■ Contaminated needles or surgical instruments ■ Mother to child at birth	■ Contaminated blood products ■ Contaminated needles ■ Intravenous (IV) drug use ■ Dialysis
Route of Infection	■ Oral ■ Fecal ■ Parenteral ■ Person to person	■ Parenteral ■ Oral ■ Fecal ■ Direct contact ■ Breast milk ■ Sexual contact	■ Parenteral ■ Sexual contact
Incubation Period	15–50 days	14–180 days	14–180 days (average)
Onset	Abrupt	Insidious	Insidious
Seasonal Variation	■ Autumn ■ Winter	All year	All year
Age Group Affected	■ Children ■ Young adults	Any age	Any age
Vaccine	Yes	Yes	No
Inoculation	Yes	Yes	Yes
Potential for Chronic Liver Disease	No	Yes	Yes
Immunity	Yes	Yes	No
Treatment	■ Prevention—hepatitis A (HAV) vaccine ■ Proper handwashing ■ Avoid contaminated food or water. ■ Obtain immunoglobulin within 14 days if exposed to the virus.	■ Prevention—hepatitis B (HBV) vaccine for high-risk groups ■ Antiviral and immunomodulating drugs	■ Subcutaneous pegylated interferon alpha once a week and oral ribavirin (Copegus, Rebetol) daily
Complications	Very few	■ Chronic hepatitis ■ Cirrhosis ■ Hepatitis D ■ Liver cancer	■ Chronic hepatitis ■ Cirrhosis ■ Liver cancer

Compare and Contrast: Parkinson's Disease, Myasthenia Gravis, and Multiple Sclerosis

	Parkinson Disease	Myasthenia Gravis	Multiple Sclerosis
Definition	Chronic, progressive neurodegenerative disorder	Autoimmune disorder of neuromuscular junction with fluctuating weakness of some skeletal muscles	Chronic, progressive, degenerative disorder Demyelination of nerve fibers of the brain and spinal cord
Patient	Peak onset in 70s, men	Onset between 10 and 65 years, women more common	Young to middle age, female, temperate climates
Etiology	Unknown but with genetic and environmental components	Antibodies attack acetylcholine receptors, which prevents stimulation of muscle contraction	Unknown; may be related to viral, immunologic, and genetic factors
Signs and Symptoms	Gradual, insidious; may be unilateral; tremor more pronounced at rest Rigidity, bradykinesia, stooped posture, drooling, masked face, shuffling gait, and jerky movements	Fluctuating weakness of skeletal muscles; strength restored after period of rest Primarily muscles of the eyes, mouth, and respiratory system Highly variable disorder	Insidious, gradual onset Remissions and exacerbations: limb weakness, diplopia, numbness, tingling, and neuropathic pain Decreased bowel, bladder function Sexual dysfunction Short-term memory and cognitive changes
Nursing Management	Maximize neurologic function Maintain independence in ADL Optimize psychosocial aspects Safety	Optimize endurance Manage fatigue Avoid complications Maintain quality of life Safety	Maintain independence in ADL Maximize neuromuscular function Manage disabling fatigue Optimize psychosocial adjustment to illness Reduce exacerbating factors Safety
Medications	Dopaminergics Anticholinergics Antihistamine Monoamine oxidase inhibitors (MAIOs) Catechol-*O*-methyltransferase (COMT) inhibitors	Anticholinesterase drugs Corticosteroids Immunosuppressants	Corticosteroids Immunomodulators Cholinergics, anticholinergics Muscle relaxants Acetylcholinesterase inhibitors

ADL, Activities of daily living.

Management/Leadership

1. **Which activity should the nurse delegate to an unlicensed assistive personnel (UAP)?**
   A. Assist a client to ambulate who was just admitted with stroke symptoms.
   B. Encourage additional oral fluids for an elderly client with pneumonia who has developed a fever.
   C. Report the ability of a client with myasthenia gravis to manage the supper tray independently.
   D. Record the number of liquid stools of a client who received lactulose for an elevated NH_3 level.

2. **The nurse is assigning tasks to the UAP. Which client situation requires the registered nurse (RN) to intervene? A client with:**
   A. active tuberculosis who is leaving the room without a mask.
   B. end-stage renal disease requesting orange juice to drink.
   C. anemia who is complaining of fatigue and asking for help getting dressed to go home.
   D. chronic obstructive pulmonary disorder who removes his oxygen and is leaving the unit to smoke.

3. **When entering a client's room, the nurse finds the client threatening to cut herself. What is the priority intervention?**
   A. Call in an extra nurse or UAP for the next shift.
   B. Assign one of the current UAPs to sit with the client.
   C. Move the client to another room with a roommate.
   D. Administer an as-needed (PRN) dose of lorazepam.

4. **A UAP is assisting with the care of several clients on a postpartum unit. Which assignment should the nurse delegate to the UAP?**
   A. Check fundal firmness and lochia for the clients who delivered vaginally.
   B. Take vital signs every 15 minutes for a client with preeclampsia.
   C. Provide breastfeeding instructions for a primigravida.
   D. Assist with daily care activities for all clients as needed.

Advanced Clinical Concepts

5. **Which client is at the highest risk for respiratory complications?**
   A. A 21-year-old client with dehydration and cerebral palsy who is dependent in daily activities.
   B. A 60-year-old client who has had type 2 diabetes for 20 years and was admitted with cellulitis.
   C. An obese 30-year-old client with hypertension who is noncompliant with the medication regimen.
   D. A 40-year-old client who takes a loop diuretic, has a serum K^+ of 3.4 mmol/L (mEq/L), and complains of fatigue.

6. **A nurse working at a clinic finds a client in one of the examination rooms slumped over and apneic. The nurse notes an empty syringe and needle still in the client's arm. Which action has the highest priority?**
   A. Call 911.
   B. Remove the syringe and needle.
   C. Assess for a pulse.
   D. Obtain the automated external defibrillator (AED).

7. **A client who is immediately postoperative for aortic aneurysm repair has been receiving normal saline intravenously at 125 mL/h. The nurse observes dark yellow urine. The hourly output for the past 3 hours was 30 mL, 18 mL, and 10 mL. What action should the nurse take?**
   A. Administer a bolus D_5 ½ normal saline at 200 mL/h.
   B. Contact the healthcare provider.
   C. Monitor output for another 2 hours.
   D. Draw blood samples for blood urea nitrogen (BUN) and creatinine levels.

8. **The RN is evaluating the effects of the administration of fresh frozen plasma (FFP) on a client diagnosed with cirrhosis. Which finding(s) would indicate a positive outcome? (Select all that apply.)**
   A. Blood urea nitrogen (BUN) 3.9 mmol/L (11 mg/dL); creatinine 62 mcmol/L (0.7 mg/dL).
   B. Hemoglobin level of 100 mmol/L (10 gm/dL).
   C. Return of temperature to normal.
   D. Decreased bleeding from the gums.
   E. Negative guaiac for occult bleeding.

9. **A client's arterial blood gas results are as follows: pH 7.29, Pco_2 55 mm Hg, and Hco_3 26 mEq/L. Which compensatory response should the nurse expect to see?**
   A. Respiratory rate of 30 breaths/min.
   B. Apical rate of 120 beats per minute.
   C. Potassium level of 5.8 mmol/L (mEq/L).
   D. Complaints of pounding headache.

10. **A client with chronic back pain is not receiving adequate pain relief from oral analgesics. Which alternative action should the nurse explore to promote the client's independence?**
   A. Ask the healthcare provider to increase the analgesic dosage.
   B. Obtain a prescription for a second analgesic to be given by the IV route.
   C. Consider the client's receptivity to complementary therapy.
   D. Encourage counseling to prevent future addiction.

Maternal/Newborn Nursing

11. **A client at 41 weeks' gestation who is in active labor calls the nurse to report that her membranes have ruptured. The nurse performs a vaginal examination and discovers that the umbilical cord has prolapsed. Which intervention should the nurse implement first?**
   A. Move the presenting fetal part off the cord.
   B. Cover the cord with sterile moist saline gauze.
   C. Prepare for an emergency cesarean delivery.
   D. Administer O_2 by face mask at 10 L/min.

12. **A client at 39 weeks' gestation plans to have an epidural block when labor is established. What intervention(s) should the nurse implement to prevent side effects? (Select all that apply.)**
   A. Teach about the procedure and effects of the epidural.
   B. Place the client in a chair next to the bed.
   C. Administer a bolus of 500 mL of normal saline solution.
   D. Monitor the fetal heart rate and contractions continuously.
   E. Assist the client to empty her bladder every 2 hours.

13. **A female client presents in the emergency department with right lower quadrant abdominal pain and pain in her right shoulder. She has no vaginal bleeding, and her last menses was 6 weeks ago. Which actions should the nurse take first?**
   A. Assess for abdominal rebound pain, distention, and fever.
   B. Obtain a complete set of vital signs and establish IV access.
   C. Observe for recent musculoskeletal injury, bruising, or abuse.
   D. Collect specimens for pregnancy test, hemoglobin, and white blood cell count.

14. **A nurse has been assigned a pregnant client who has heart disease. The client's condition has been diagnosed as New York Heart Association (NYHA) class II cardiac disease. What important fact(s) about activities of daily living while pregnant should the nurse teach this client? (Select all that apply.)**
   A. Increase fiber in the diet.
   B. Anticipate the need for rest breaks after activity.
   C. Notify the healthcare provider if her rings do not fit.
   D. Maintain bed rest with bathroom privileges.
   E. Start a low-impact aerobic exercise program.

Medical-Surgical

15. **A client with type II diabetes is scheduled for an intravenous pyelogram (IVP). Which assessment is most important for the nurse to complete before the test is performed?**
   a. Baseline vital signs.
   b. Current medication list.
   c. Coagulation status.
   d. Electrolyte levels.

16. **The nurse is teaching a client who has chronic urinary tract infections about a prescription for ciprofloxacin 500 mg PO bid (twice daily). What side effect(s) could the client expect while taking this medication? (Select all that apply.)**
   A. Photosensitivity.
   B. Dyspepsia.
   C. Diarrhea.
   D. Urinary frequency.
   E. Anemia.

17. **An RN working on a hospice unit finds a client crying. The client states that he is afraid to die. Which actions should the RN implement? (Select all that apply.)**
   A. Sit quietly with the client and listen to his concerns.
   B. Provide the client with privacy.
   C. Give the client an antianxiety medication.
   D. Contact the client's spiritual counselor or pastor.
   E. Assess the patient for signs of impending death.

18. **A male client with a peritoneal dialysis (PD) catheter calls the clinic to report that he feels poorly and has a fever. What is the best response by the nurse?**
   A. Encourage him to come to the clinic today for assessment.
   B. Instruct him to increase his fluid intake to 3 L/day.
   C. Review his peritoneal dialysis regimen.
   D. Inquire about his recent dietary intake of protein and iron.

19. The nurse is reviewing the cardiac markers for a client who was admitted with the diagnosis of chest pain. Which marker is the best to determine cardiac damage?
   A. Troponin levels.
   B. Myoglobin level.
   C. Creatine kinase myocardial band (CK-MB) level.
   D. Lactate dehydrogenase (LDH) level.

20. The nurse is providing discharge instructions to a client who has been diagnosed with angina pectoris. Which instruction is most important?
   A. Avoid activity that involves the Valsalva maneuver.
   B. Seek emergency treatment if chest pain persists after the third nitroglycerin dose.
   C. Rest for 30 minutes after having chest pain before resuming activity.
   D. Keep extra nitroglycerin in an airtight, light-resistant bottle.

21. The nurse is providing discharge teaching for a client who has been prescribed diltiazem. Which dietary instruction has the highest priority?
   A. Maintain a low-sodium diet.
   B. Eat a banana each morning.
   C. Ingest high-fiber foods daily.
   D. Avoid grapefruit products.

22. The nurse is teaching a young adult female who has a history of Raynaud disease how to control her pain. What information should the nurse offer?
   A. Take oral analgesics at regularly spaced intervals.
   B. Avoid extremes of heat and cold.
   C. Limit foods and fluids that contain caffeine.
   D. Keep the affected extremities in a dependent position.

23. The clinic nurse is caring for a client taking argatroban for atrial fibrillation. What information is essential for the nurse to include in the client's teaching plan? (Select all that apply.)
   A. Have protamine sulfate available.
   B. Notify the healthcare provider of any unusual bleeding.
   C. Eat a diet high in green leafy vegetables.
   D. Keep the medication in a dark, dry container.
   E. Avoid aspirin or aspirin-containing medications.

24. A client who was admitted to the hospital with cancer of the larynx is scheduled for a laryngectomy tomorrow. What is the client's priority learning need tonight?
   A. Anticipated body image changes.
   B. Pain management expectations.
   C. Communication techniques.
   D. Postoperative nutritional needs.

Psychiatric Nursing

25. A victim of a motor vehicle collision is dead on arrival at the emergency department. The significant other arrives and is noticeably upset. What action should the nurse take to assist the significant other with this crisis?
   A. Ask whether there are family, friends, or clergy to call.
   B. Talk about the former relationship with the significant other.
   C. Provide education about the stages of grief and loss.
   D. Assess the significant other's level of anxiety.

26. The nurse is planning to lead a seminar for community health nurses on violence against women during pregnancy. Which statement describes an appropriate technique for assessing for violence?
   A. Women should be assessed only if they are part of a high-risk group.
   B. Women may be assessed in the presence of young children but not intimate partners.
   C. The assessment only needs to be completed at the beginning of the pregnancy.
   D. Women should be reassessed face-to-face by a nurse as the pregnancy progresses.

27. The charge nurse reminds clients on the mental health unit that breakfast is at 8 AM, medications are given at 9 AM, and group therapy sessions begin at 10 AM. Which treatment modality has been implemented?
   A. Milieu therapy.
   B. Behavior modification.
   C. Peer therapy.
   D. Problem-solving.

28. The nurse is accompanying a client to the radiography department when he becomes panic stricken at the elevator and states, "I can't get on that elevator." Which action should the nurse take first?
   A. Ask one more staff member to ride in the elevator.
   B. Offer a prescribed antianxiety medication.
   C. Begin desensitization about riding the elevator.
   D. Affirm the client's fears about riding the elevator.

29. A client who has posttraumatic stress disorder is found one night trying to strangle his roommate. Which intervention is the nurse's highest priority?
   A. Give the client a sedative or hypnotic.
   B. Administer an antipsychotic.
   C. Assign a UAP to sit with the client.
   D. Process with both clients about event.

30. The nurse is updating the plan of care for a client who has a borderline personality disorder. Which intervention is most important to implement?
    A. Assign the same nurse to care for the client.
    B. Avoid challenging inappropriate behavior.
    C. Limit the client's contact with other clients.
    D. Remove consequences for acting-out behaviors.

31. A female adolescent is admitted to the mental health unit for anorexia nervosa. In planning care, what is the nurse's highest priority?
    A. Teach the client the importance of self-expression.
    B. Supervise the client's activities closely.
    C. Include the client in daily group therapy.
    D. Facilitate social interactions with others.

32. The charge nurse is planning the daily schedule for clients on the mental health unit. A male client who is manic should be assigned to which activity?
    A. A basketball game in the gym.
    B. Jogging at least 1 mile daily.
    C. A table tennis game with a peer.
    D. Group activity with the art therapist.

Leadership and Delegation

33. A nurse is planning the client assignments for the night shift. The nursing team includes a registered nurse, a licensed practical nurse, and two unlicensed assistive personnel (UAP). Which duty (or duties) could be delegated to the UAPs? (Select all that apply.)
    A. Transport a client to the radiology department for a computed tomography (CT) scan.
    B. Bathe a client with sickle cell disease who has multiple IV lines and a patient-controlled analgesia pump.
    C. Turn a 92-year-old client who has end-stage heart failure and a do-not-resuscitate order.
    D. Report to the healthcare provider the fingerstick blood glucose level of 2.72 mmol/L (49 mg/dL)
    E. Feed a female client her first meal after she experienced a stroke.

34. A hospitalized client has been newly diagnosed with type 2 diabetes. Which task(s) can the RN delegate to the UAP? (Select all that apply.)
    A. Contacting the dietitian for a prescribed consult.
    B. Reviewing the client's insulin injection technique.
    C. Obtaining the fingerstick blood glucose level before each meal and at bedtime.
    D. Reminding the client to dry the toes carefully after a shower.
    E. Talking to the client about foods that raise the blood glucose level.

35. The home health nurse evaluates the insulin preparation and administration technique of a 36-year-old male client newly diagnosed with diabetes. The client has been prescribed lispro insulin before meals and glargine insulin once daily in the morning. Which finding indicates that the client needs further education?
    A. He mixes glargine and lispro in the same syringe for the morning dose.
    B. He leaves the insulin syringe in place for 10 seconds after injection.
    C. He stores the opened insulin vials at room temperature in the cabinet.
    D. He recaps and disposes of the single-use insulin syringe.

36. At change of shift, the charge nurse assigns the UAP four clients. The RN should direct the UAP to take vital signs on which client first?
    A. The 89-year-old with chronic obstructive pulmonary disease who is resting quietly on 2 L of oxygen and who needs assistance with a bath.
    B. The client who returned from surgery and needs their second set of every-15-minute vitals signs taken.
    C. The client newly diagnosed with type 2 diabetes who had a fingerstick glucose level of 5.0 mmol/L (90 mg/dL) and needs help with breakfast.
    D. The newly admitted client with rheumatoid arthritis who needs hand splints reapplied to both hands.

37. The arrythmia alarm sounds on a client on the telemetry unit, indicating that the client is in ventricular tachycardia. Place the nurse's actions for this client in order of priority from first to last.
    A. Call the rapid responses team.
    B. Assess for blood pressure.
    C. Give oxygen via nasal cannula.
    D. Bring defibrillator/crash car to the bedside.
    E. Document the incident.

38. The nurse is reviewing the laboratory values of her assigned clients. Which client has an abnormal laboratory report that the nurse should immediately call to the healthcare provider?
    A. The client who is post splenectomy after a motor vehicle accident and has a hemoglobin of 109 mmol/L (10.9 g/dL).
    B. The client receiving warfarin (Coumadin) who has an international normalized ratio (INR) of 2.3.
    C. The 38-year-old client who is 24 hours postthyroidectomy and has a total calcium level of 2.35 mmol/L (9.4 mg/dL).
    D. The newly admitted client with bipolar disorder with a lithium level of 2.5 mEq/L.

39. The nurse receives change-of-shift report on her four acute care clients. Which action should the nurse take first?
   A. Administer an antiemetic to a postoperative client who has been nauseated and is now vomiting.
   B. Notify a family member of a client's impending transfer to the intensive care unit for angina and ST segment changes.
   C. Inform the healthcare provider of a potassium level of 5.2 mmol/L (mEq/L) in the client with end-stage renal disease.
   D. Begin assessment rounds, starting with the palliative care client having a diagnosis of congestive failure.

40. The emergency department staff nurse is assigned four clients. Which client should the nurse assess first?
   A. A preschooler with a barking cough, an O_2 saturation of 93% on room air, and occasional inspiratory stridor.
   B. A 10-month-old infant with a tympanic temperature of 38.9°C (102°F) and green nasal drainage who is pulling at her ears.
   C. A crying 8-month-old with a harsh, paroxysmal cough; an audible expiratory wheeze; and mild retractions.
   D. A clingy 3-year-old who has a sore throat and drooling and whose tongue is slightly protruding from his mouth.

41. The outpatient clinic nurse is reviewing phone messages from the previous night. Which client should the nurse call back first?
   A. A woman at 30 weeks' gestation who has been diagnosed with mild preeclampsia and was unable to relieve her heartburn.
   B. A woman at 24 weeks' gestation who was crying about painful vulvar lesions and urinary frequency for the past 8 hours.
   C. A woman at 12 weeks' gestation who was recently discharged from the hospital with hyperemesis gravidarum and had had two episodes of vomiting in 6 hours.
   D. A woman with type 1 diabetes who tested positive with a home pregnancy kit and was worried about managing her diabetes.

42. The clinic nurse suspects that a 2-year-old child is being abused. Which assessment finding(s) would support this? (Select all that apply.)
   A. Petechiae in a straight line on the chest.
   B. Gray-blue pigmented areas on the sacral region.
   C. Bald patches on the scalp.
   D. Ear tugging and crying.
   E. Symmetrical burns on the hands.

43. The nurse is caring for a client who had a thoracotomy 48 hours earlier and has left lower lobe chest tubes. The nurse notes that a chest tube is not tidaling. Which action should the nurse take first?
   A. Check for kinks in the chest drainage system.
   B. Assess the heart rate and blood pressure.
   C. Notify the rapid response team immediately.
   D. Reconnect the chest tube to wall suction.

44. While the nurse is caring for a client who has had a myocardial infarction, the monitor alarm sounds, and the nurse notes ventricular fibrillation. What should be the nurse's first course of action?
   A. Notify the healthcare provider.
   B. Increase the oxygen concentration.
   C. Assess the client.
   D. Prepare to defibrillate the client.

45. The healthcare provider has prescribed the removal of a client's internal jugular central line catheter. To remove the catheter safely, the nurse should give which intervention(s) the highest priority? (Select all that apply.)
   A. Carefully remove the bio-occlusive dressing.
   B. Place the client in the Trendelenburg position.
   C. Send the catheter tip to the laboratory for a culture and sensitivity.
   D. Have the client hold a deep breath during removal.
   E. Apply pressure for 20 minutes after removal of the catheter.

46. The nurse who usually works on the orthopedic surgery unit is floating to a cardiovascular unit. Which client would be best to assign to the float nurse?
   A. Client scheduled for a heart catheterization this morning.
   B. Client admitted last night for chest pain.
   C. Client who is 1 day postoperative for popliteal bypass surgery.
   D. Client with heart failure and scheduled for a stress test today.

47. The nurse is admitting a client who is a paraplegic and has a nonhealing pressure injury with a possible methicillin-resistant *Staphylococcus aureus* infection. A PN and UAP are assigned to the nurse's team. Which tasks should be delegated to the PN? (Select all that apply.)
   A. Place the client in isolation.
   B. Complete a dressing change.
   C. Assess and document the wound.
   D. Insert a urinary catheter.
   E. Administer oral pain medications.

48. The nursing supervisor calls the charge nurse on a step-down unit about the need for a bed for an unstable patient from the medical unit. Which client should the nurse transfer to the medical unit to receive this unstable client?
A. A client admitted for an ST-elevation myocardial infarction (STEMI) who just returned from having a cardiac catheterization performed.
B. A client diagnosed with congestive heart failure who is receiving an IV infusion of furosemide.
C. A client with possible Guillain-Barré syndrome who may need an exchange transfusion.
D. A client in hypertensive crisis who is prescribed a sodium nitroprusside drip.

49. When accessing the medication dispensing system (Pyxis), the nurse finds chlorpropamide in the drawer instead of the expected chlorpromazine. Which actions should the nurse take? (Select all that apply.)
A. Remove the tablets of chlorpropamide.
B. Notify the pharmacy about the mistake.
C. Place an incident occurrence report.
D. Be extra vigilant because pharmacy is making mistakes.
E. Place a warning note on the Pyxis machine.

50. The nurse is calling the healthcare provider (HCP) about a client's current needs. What is the best way to communicate?
A. Call the HCP with the request and a recommendation.
B. Use the SBAR (situation, background, assessment, recommendation) tool for communication.
C. Send a text message or page with the needed order.
D. Ask the HCP to come back to the unit to discuss the client's needs.

51. The healthcare provider plans to do a paracentesis on a client with cirrhosis in 1 hour. In what order should the nurse perform the following activities?
A. Ensure that the informed consent has been obtained.
B. Measure the client's abdominal girth.
C. Have the client empty his or her bladder.
D. Assemble needed equipment.
E. Administer oral pain medication.

52. The nurse receives report on a client from the emergency department with a diagnosis of pneumonia. Which intervention has the highest priority?
A. Obtain blood cultures.
B. Initiate prescribed antibiotics.
C. Place the client in isolation.
D. Obtain an accurate weight.

53. The nurse is part of the triage team at a disaster. Which client should be seen first?
A. A 90-year-old woman with a crushed pelvis and head injuries.
B. A 21-year-old man screaming in pain from a broken leg.
C. A 30-year-old woman with a flail chest secondary to a puncture wound to the chest.
D. A 12-year-old crying with multiple lacerations to both legs.

54. The triage nurse in the emergency room is assessing four clients. Which client requires the most immediate intervention?
A. The adult client who arrived via ambulance with numbness and tingling of his left arm and face.
B. The adult client who had a seizure at home who is sleeping on his left side.
C. The 60-year-old client who complains of frequent urination and has a blood sugar of 16.7 mmol/L (300 mg/dL).
D. The middle-aged client who presents with severe unilateral back pain and previous history of kidney stones.

55. After a change-of-shift report on an orthopedic floor, which client should the nurse assess first?
A. A client who had surgery yesterday and has a temperature of 37.6°C (99.7°F).
B. A client who is complaining of numbness and tingling distal to the fracture site.
C. A client who had a left leg amputation and states he is experiencing pain in the left foot.
D. A client who is extremely upset with their care and is requesting to speak to the manager.

56. The nurse is administering medications to a client admitted for an overdose and a history of substance abuse. Which intervention(s) is (are) a priority to include in this client's plan of care? (Select all that apply.)
A. Allow the client to take medications independently.
B. Ensure that all medications have been swallowed before leaving the client's room.
C. Request that oral pain medications be changed from tablet to oral suspension.
D. Administer flumazenil as prescribed every 6 hours around the clock.
E. Administer all medications to the client via the intravenous route.

57. The nurse is returning phone calls to clients who are cared for at an outpatient mental health center. Which client should the nurse call first?
A. The young mother diagnosed with schizophrenia who is hearing voices saying that they are pursuing her children.

B. The elderly man at an assisted living facility who says he wants to end it all.

C. The female client diagnosed with bipolar disorder who has not slept for 48 hours.

D. The teenager diagnosed with bulimia whose mother called and reported that she found her daughter purging.

58. **An 18-year-old woman is being discharged after delivering a healthy baby. She has a cousin whose baby died from sudden infant death syndrome (SIDS). The client seems to know many of the precautions to take. Which information does the nurse need to correct?**
A. Always place infants on their backs to sleep.
B. Room sharing has been shown to decrease SIDS.
C. Keep the crib free of stuffed animals and crib pads.
D. Sleeping with the baby can alert the mother to changes.

59. **A 4-year-old admitted with pneumonia weighs 18 kg. The healthcare provider has prescribed vancomycin 40 mg/kg/day IV. The order states to divide the dose and give it three times daily. How many milligrams of vancomycin should the child receive in each dose? (Round the answer to the nearest whole number.)**

_____ mg/dose

60. **The nurse needs to initiate an IV on an 8-year-old child. Which intervention(s) is/are appropriate?**
A. Start the IV in the treatment room, not the child's room.
B. Apply a lidocaine-based cream for a few minutes before starting the IV.
C. Ask the parents to leave the room while performing the procedure.
D. Encourage the child to use guided imagery to cope.
E. Offer the child a reward if they cooperate during the procedure.

Answers and Rationales

(Correct answers are underlined.)

Management/Leadership

1. **Which activity should the nurse delegate to an unlicensed assistive personnel (UAP)?**
Rationales:
A. *Assist a client to ambulate who was just admitted with stroke symptoms.*
This requires assessment of the client's ability to ambulate safely, which is beyond the scope of practice of a UAP.
B. *Encourage additional PO (by mouth) fluids for an elderly client with pneumonia who has developed a fever.*

These directions are not sufficiently clear and detailed for the UAP to perform the task.
C. ***Report the ability of a client with myasthenia gravis to manage the supper tray independently.***
This requires assessment of the client's clinical status, which is beyond the scope of the UAP.
D. ***Record the number of liquid stools of a client who has received lactulose for an increased NH3 level.***
This task encompasses basic care, elimination, and intake and output; it does not require judgment or the expertise of the nurse and can be performed by the UAP.

2. **The nurse is assigning tasks to the UAP. Which client situation requires the RN to intervene? A client with:**
Rationales:
A. *active TB who is leaving the room without a mask.*
A UAP can be delegated to provide a box of masks or to direct the client back to the room.
B. ***end-stage renal disease requesting orange juice to drink.***
A UAP can be directed to provide specific types and amounts of fluids, but orange juice is high in potassium, which is contraindicated for patients in end-stage renal disease.
C. *anemia who is complaining of fatigue and asking for help getting dressed to go home.*
A UAP can assist a client to get dressed. Fatigue is an expected finding with anemia.
D. *chronic obstructive pulmonary disorder removes his oxygen and is leaving the unit to smoke.*
A UAP can ask the client to not leave the unit to smoke.

3. **When entering a client's room, the nurse finds the client threatening to cut herself. What is the priority intervention?**
Rationales:
A. *Call in an extra nurse or UAP for the next shift.*
The charge nurse should plan ahead for staffing, but the immediate focus should be the client's safety now.
B. ***Assign one of the current UAPs to sit with the client.***
Because the client is at risk for self-harm, the charge nurse should assign a staff member to stay with the client.
C. *Move the client to another room with a roommate.*
This will not ensure the client's safety; also, a staff member, not another client, must always be present with the client.
D. *Administer an as-needed (PRN) dose of lorazepam as prescribed.*
Although the client may be anxious, this is not a priority intervention that would ensure her safety.

4. A UAP is assisting with the care of several clients on a postpartum unit. Which assignment should the nurse delegate to the UAP?

Rationales:

A. *Check fundal firmness and lochia for the clients who delivered vaginally.*
Assessment is a responsibility of the nurse.

B. *Take vital signs every 15 minutes for a client with preeclampsia.*
This is a high-risk patient who needs to be evaluated by a licensed nurse.

C. *Provide breastfeeding instructions for a primigravida.*
Teaching is the responsibility of the RN.

D. *Assist with daily care activities for all clients as needed.*
This is the most appropriate assignment for the UAP. The RN should delegate daily care activities to the UAP based on the RN's assessments of each client's needs.

Advanced Clinical Concepts

5. Which client is at the highest risk for respiratory complications?

Rationales:

A. *A 21-year-old client with dehydration and cerebral palsy who is dependent in daily activities.*
A client with dehydration and cerebral palsy, characterized by uncoordinated, spastic muscle movements, is at increased risk for respiratory problems because of impaired mobility and impaired swallowing.

B. *A 60-year-old client who has had type 2 diabetes for 20 years and was admitted with cellulitis.*
This older client is more at risk for renal, cardiac, and vascular complications.

C. *An obese 30-year-old client with hypertension who is noncompliant with the medication regimen.*
An obese adult who is noncompliant with antihypertensive medications is more at risk for cardiac or cerebral events than for respiratory problems.

D. *A 40-year-old client who takes a loop diuretic, has a serum K^+ of 3.4 mmol/L (mEq/L), and complains of fatigue.*
This middle-aged adult is hypokalemic and fatigued but is not at high risk for respiratory problems.

6. A nurse working at a clinic finds a client in one of the examination rooms slumped over and apneic. The nurse notes an empty syringe and needle still in the client's arm. Which action has the highest priority?

Rationales:

A. *Call 911.*
Calling for assistance is a high priority but not the highest.

B. *Remove the syringe and needle.*
The syringe and needle should be removed and possibly sent to a laboratory for analysis of the contents, but this is not a priority.

C. *Assess for a pulse.*
Assessing for a pulse is the highest priority to determine whether cardiopulmonary resuscitation (CPR) needs to be initiated.

D. *Obtain the AED.*
This action is needed only if there is no pulse detected.

7. A client who is immediately postoperative for abdominal aortic aneurysm repair has been receiving normal saline intravenously at 125 mL/hr. The nurse observes dark yellow urine. The hourly output for the past 3 hours was 30 mL, 18 mL, and 10mL. What action should the nurse take?

Rationales:

A. *Administer a bolus D_5 ½ normal saline at 200 mL/hr.*
The decreasing urine output may be a sign of acute renal failure, a complication of aortic aneurysm repair. Giving more fluids may cause the client's condition to deteriorate.

B. *Contact the healthcare provider.*
Acute renal failure can result from interruption of blood flow during an aortic aneurysm repair. Low urinary output may indicate acute renal failure and requires more immediate intervention from the healthcare provider.

C. *Monitor output for another 2 hours.*
Urine output has been monitored, and further intervention is needed.

D. *Draw blood samples for blood urea nitrogen (BUN) and creatinine levels.*
The BUN and creatinine should be evaluated, but these tests are not the immediate priority.

8. The RN is evaluating the effects of the administration of fresh frozen plasma (FFP) on a client diagnosed with cirrhosis. Which finding(s) would indicate a positive outcome? (Select all that apply.)

Rationales:

A. *Blood urea nitrogen (BUN) 3.9 mmol/L (11 mg/dL); creatinine 62 mcmol/L (0.7 mg/dL).*
These values are not affected by administration of FFP. They assess renal function.

B. *Hemoglobin level of 100 mmol/L (10 gm/dL).*
FFP does not affect hemoglobin levels.

C. *Return of temperature to normal.*
Although monitoring the client's temperature is important, FFP does not have a direct effect on this parameter.

D. *Decreased bleeding from the gums.*
FFP replaces clotting factors; therefore, a decrease in bleeding is an expected, positive outcome.

E. *Negative guaiac for occult bleeding.*

FFP replaces clotting factors; therefore, no occult (hidden) bleeding would be an expected, positive outcome.

9. **A client's arterial blood gas results are as follows: pH 7.29, Pco2 55 mm Hg, and Hco3 26 mEq/L. Which compensatory response should the nurse expect to see?**
Rationales:
   A. *Respiratory rate of 30 breaths/min.*
   The client is experiencing respiratory acidosis. In addition to the metabolic system compensating, the respiratory system may also compensate.
   B. *Apical rate of 120 beat per minute.*
   Acid-base imbalances are compensated primarily by the lungs and the renal system. Plasma proteins and ionic shifts (intracellular) also serve as buffering systems. Tachycardia does not serve as a compensatory mechanism.
   C. *Potassium level of 5.8 mmol/L (mEq/L).*
   To compensate for the acidosis created by increased CO_2, K^+ ions are released from cellular proteins and H^+ ions take their place, bound to the proteins. The result is frequently serum hyperkalemia.
   D. *Complaints of a pounding headache.*
   Headache may be a manifestation of CO_2 retention, but it is not a compensatory mechanism for respiratory acidosis.

10. **A client with chronic back pain is not receiving adequate pain relief from oral analgesics. Which alternative action should the nurse explore to promote the client's independence?**
Rationales:
   A. *Ask the healthcare provider to increase the analgesic dosage.*
   Although this intervention may improve pain relief, it may not promote self-care without increasing side effects that could affect the client's independence.
   B. *Obtain a prescription for a second analgesic to be given by the IV route.*
   The IV route does not promote self-care and may cause additional side effects that interfere with the client's ability to carry out activities of daily living independently.
   C. *Consider the client's receptivity to complementary therapy.*
   This action supports self-care without the high level of adverse effects associated with additional medication. It is the least invasive measure, and it promotes the active participation (self-care) of the client.
   D. *Encourage counseling to prevent future addiction.*
   Referrals may be needed, but the nurse should teach clients about potential problems with medications and measures to manage pain and maintain self-care.

Maternal-Newborn Nursing

11. **A client at 41 weeks' gestation who is in active labor calls the nurse to report that her membranes have ruptured. The nurse performs a vaginal examination and discovers that the umbilical cord has prolapsed. Which intervention should the nurse implement first?**
Rationales:
   A. *Move the presenting fetal part off the cord.*
   This action is the most critical intervention. The nurse must prevent compression of the cord by the presenting part because that would impair fetal circulation, leading to morbidity and, possibly, death.
   B. *Cover the cord with sterile moist saline gauze.*
   If the cord is protruding outside the vagina, this action should be taken to prevent drying of the Wharton's jelly. However, another nurse should do this while the first nurse maintains elevation of the presenting part off the cord.
   C. *Prepare for an emergency cesarean delivery.*
   This is implemented by the staff while the nurse keeps the presenting part elevated off the cord.
   D. *Start O_2 by face mask at 10 L/min.*
   Oxygen should be provided to the mother to increase oxygen delivery to the fetus via the placenta; however, another nurse should do this while first the nurse keeps the presenting part elevated off the cord.

12. **A client at 39 weeks' gestation plans to have an epidural block when labor is established. What intervention(s) should the nurse be prepared to implement to prevent side effects? (Select all that apply.)**
Rationales:
   A. *Teach the client about the procedure and the effects of the epidural.*
   Teaching is an important nursing intervention to alleviate anxiety, but it does not prevent any of the possible side effects.
   B. *Place the client in a chair next to the bed.*
   Epidural block reduces lower extremity sensation and movement to varying degrees. Any upright positions such as walking and standing may not be possible during epidural pain management and may not prevent side effects.
   C. *Administer a bolus of 500 mL of normal saline solution.*
   Prehydration increases maternal blood volume and prevents hypotension, which occurs as a result of vasodilation, a side effect of epidural anesthesia. A saline solution is used to prevent fetal secretion of insulin that later places the neonate at risk for hypoglycemia.
   D. *Monitor the fetal heart rate and contractions continuously.*
   Vital signs should be monitored every 5 minutes immediately after the initial epidural dose, and if the client's condition is stable, then every 15 minutes.

E. *Assist the client to empty her bladder every 2 hours.*
Assisting the client to void every 2 hours prevents bladder distention.

13. **A female client presents in the emergency department with right lower quadrant abdominal pain and pain in her right shoulder. She has no vaginal bleeding, and her last menses was 6 weeks ago. Which actions should the nurse take first?**
Rationales:
    A. *Assess for abdominal rebound pain, distention, and fever.*
    Bleeding related to an ectopic pregnancy (based on the client's history) may present these manifestations, but the nurse should first assess the client for early signs of hypovolemic shock.
    B. *Obtain a complete set of vital signs and establish IV access.*
    The nurse should first evaluate the client for vital sign changes related to blood loss due to a possible ruptured ectopic pregnancy (an obstetrical emergency). Vascular access is vital in an emergency situation.
    C. *Observe for recent musculoskeletal injury, bruising, or abuse.*
    This may be part of the assessment if a life-threatening situation is ruled out first.
    D. *Collect specimens for pregnancy test, hemoglobin, and white blood cell count.*
    Specimens for a pregnancy test and complete blood count should be collected. However, the nurse should first notify the healthcare provider of the client's status, based on the presenting vital signs and symptoms.

14. **A nurse has been assigned a pregnant client who has heart disease. The client's condition has been diagnosed as New York Heart Association (NYHA) class II cardiac disease. What important fact(s) about activities of daily living while pregnant should the nurse teach this client? (Select all that apply.)**
Rationales:
    A. *Increase fiber in the diet.*
    Restrictions in activities of daily living for clients with NYHA Class II cardiac disease create a risk factor for constipation.
    B. *Anticipate the need for rest breaks after activity.*
    Individuals with NYHA Class II cardiac disease may have limitations on activity and need periods of rest throughout the day, but especially after periods of activity.
    C. *Notify the healthcare provider if her rings do not fit.*
    Tight rings may indicate weight gain, and the client is at risk for congestive heart failure.
    D. *Maintain bed rest with bathroom privileges.*
    It is not necessary to maintain bed rest for a client with NYHA Class II cardiac disease.

E. *Start a low-impact aerobic exercise program.*
Individuals with NYHA class II cardiac disease may have some slight limitation of activity. Additionally, during pregnancy is not an ideal time to start a new exercise program.

Medical-Surgical:

15. **A client with type II diabetes is scheduled for an intravenous pyelogram (IVP). Which assessment is most important for the nurse to complete before the test is performed?**
Rationales:
    A. *Baseline vital signs.*
    Baseline values are important but there is a higher priority.
    B. *Current medication list.*
    This is a priority. If the client is taking an oral diabetic agent with metformin, the nurse may need to hold the medication for 48 hours before the IVP because of potentially decreased kidney function.
    C. *Coagulation status.*
    There is no risk of bleeding related to an IVP.
    D. *Electrolyte levels.*
    Electrolyte levels are not affected by an IVP, and high or low levels are not considered a contraindication for completing the test.

16. **The nurse is teaching a client who has chronic urinary tract infections about a prescription for ciprofloxacin 500 mg PO bid (twice daily). What side effect(s) could the client expect while taking this medication? (Select all that apply.)**
Rationales:
    A. *Photosensitivity.*
    This is a side effect of ciprofloxacin; exposure to sunlight or tanning beds should be avoided. The client should be instructed to use sunscreen and protective clothing.
    B. *Dyspepsia.*
    Ciprofloxacin causes gastrointestinal irritation, nausea and vomiting, and abdominal pain, which should be reported.
    C. *Diarrhea.*
    Watery, foul-smelling diarrhea is an adverse reaction to ciprofloxacin that indicates pseudomembranous colitis; this should be reported and requires immediate intervention.
    D. *Urinary frequency.*
    Urinary frequency may indicate that the medication is ineffective and should be reported, but it is not an expected side effect.
    E. *Anemia.*
    This is not a side effect of ciprofloxacin.

17. **An RN working on a hospice unit finds a client crying. The client states that he is afraid to die. Which actions should the RN implement? (Select all that apply).**

A. *Sit quietly with the client and listen to his concerns.*
Silence, or offering one's presence, is an effective technique that lets the client share as he desires and also indicates that the nurse cares.

B. *Provide the client with privacy.*
The client has shared that he is afraid. Further isolating the patient from others will not address this need.

C. *Give the client an antianxiety medication.*
The nurse may eventually decide to give the client a medication to help with his anxiety, but this should not be the first action.

D. *Contact the client's spiritual counselor or minister.*
Facing death is a spiritual issue. Requesting help from the client's spiritual provider is appropriate.

E. *Assess the patient for signs of impending death.*
The client is awake and oriented. There is no indication that the client's death is imminent.

18. **A male client with a peritoneal dialysis (PD) catheter calls the clinic to report he feels poorly and has a fever. What is the best response by the nurse?**
    Rationales:

    A. *Encourage him to come to the clinic today for assessment.*
    PD catheters are used in peritoneal dialysis. They are often used at home by the client, placing the client at risk for peritoneal infection. Because dialysis clients usually have some degree of compromised immunity, the client should come to the clinic for assessment.

    B. *Instruct him to increase his fluid intake to 3 L/day.*
    Clients who need dialysis retain fluid and usually are restricted to an intake that is only 300 mL greater than output.

    C. *Review his peritoneal dialysis regimen.*
    The nurse should evaluate the client's peritoneal dialysis regimen, but assessing him for infection is a higher priority.

    D. *Inquire about his recent dietary intake of protein and iron.*
    Iron deficiency and protein loss are common problems in clients who are receiving peritoneal dialysis. Dietary intake is important, but it is not a higher priority than possible infection.

19. **The nurse is reviewing the cardiac markers for a client who was admitted with the diagnosis of chest pain. Which marker is the best to determine cardiac damage?**
    Rationales:

    A. *Troponin levels.*

    A rise in the troponin levels is diagnostic of myocardial injury and is considered the gold standard.

    B. *Myoglobin level.*
    An increase in myoglobin is indicative of muscle damage but is not specific to cardiac damage.

    C. *Creatine kinase myocardial band (CK-MB) level.*
    This isoenzyme is useful for supporting a diagnosis of myocardial infarction and in determining the extent and time of the infarct.

    D. *Lactate dehydrogenase (LDH) level.*
    The LDH level is not currently used to determine recent cardiac damage.

20. **The nurse is providing discharge instructions to a client who has been diagnosed with angina pectoris. Which instruction is most important?**
    Rationales:

    A. *Avoid activity that involves the Valsalva maneuver.*
    Although minimizing or avoiding the Valsalva maneuver decreases anginal pain, this is not the most important factor.

    B. *Seek emergency treatment if chest pain persists after the third nitroglycerin dose.*
    This instruction is most important because chest pain characteristic of acute myocardial infarction persists longer than 15 minutes, and delaying medical treatment can be life-threatening.

    C. *Rest for 30 minutes after having chest pain before resuming activity.*
    Waiting 30 minutes may be recommended, but the need to call 911 if chest pain persists is more important.

    D. *Keep extra nitroglycerin in an airtight, light-resistant bottle.*
    This is excellent medication teaching, but it does not have the same urgency as seeking emergency care.

21. **The nurse is providing discharge teaching for a client who has been prescribed diltiazem. Which dietary instruction has the highest priority?**
    Rationales:

    A. *Maintain a low-sodium diet.*
    The client may need to restrict sodium intake, but it is not specific for diltiazem.

    B. *Eat a banana each morning.*
    If the client has low potassium, this should be recommended.

    C. *Ingest high-fiber foods daily.*
    This is an excellent teaching point for everyone, but it is not specific for diltiazem.

    D. *Avoid grapefruit products.*
    Grapefruit should be avoided during therapy with calcium channel blockers because it can cause an increase in the serum drug level, predisposing the client to hypotension.

22. **The nurse is teaching a young adult female who has a history of Raynaud disease how to control her pain. What information should the nurse offer?**
Rationales:
A. *Take oral analgesics at regularly spaced intervals.*
Pain is not always associated with Raynaud disease as is the feeling of cold hands and fingers and pallor. If pain is sporadic or situational, it should not require regular use of analgesics.
B. *Avoid extremes of heat and cold.*
In Raynaud disease, vascular spasms of the hands and fingers are triggered by exposure to extremes of heat or cold, which causes the characteristic pallor and cold-to-the-touch symptoms of the upper extremities.
C. *Limit food and fluids that contain caffeine.*
Caffeine is not the primary trigger of the episodes; however, if the client notes that caffeine contributes to the blanching and coldness, it should be avoided.
D. *Keep the affected extremities in a dependent position.*
This is not effective for a client with Raynaud disease.

23. **The nurse is caring for a client taking argatroban for atrial fibrillation. What information is essential for the nurse to include in the client's teaching plan? (Select all that apply.)**
Rationales:
A. *Have protamine sulfate available.*
Protamine sulfate is the antidote for heparin, not argatroban.
B. *Notify the healthcare provider of any unusual bleeding.*
Gastrointestinal (GI) bleeding or excessive bleeding is an adverse effect. The client needs to notify their healthcare provider immediately.
C. *Eat a diet high in green leafy vegetables.*
This is a good recommendation for clients low in vitamin K but is not an issue for clients on argatroban.
D. *Keep the medication in a dark, dry container.*
This is essential for nitroglycerin and some other medications but not for argatroban.
E. *Avoid aspirin or aspirin-containing medications*
Aspirin and argatroban can have an additive effect and result in bleeding.

24. **A client who was admitted to the hospital with cancer of the larynx is scheduled for a laryngectomy tomorrow. What is the client's priority learning need tonight?**
Rationales:
A. *Anticipated body image changes.*
This is a concern after surgery, when the immediate life-threatening insult of cancer has been assimilated and basic needs have been met.
B. *Pain management expectations.*
Pain relief expectations are a priority, but the inability to convey (communicate) a subjective symptom, such as pain, is the fear the client perceives first.
C. *Communication techniques.*
A client who is in crisis and anticipating the immediate postoperative period is concerned with immediate needs, such as the ability to express and convey a subjective symptom (e.g., pain) and obtain the needed intervention.
D. *Postoperative nutritional needs.*
Nutrition is important to promote healing, but the ability to communicate subjective needs is a higher priority.

Psychiatric Nursing

25. **A victim of a motor vehicle collision is dead on arrival at the emergency department. The victim's significant other arrives and is noticeably upset. What action should the nurse implement to assist the significant other?**
Rationales:
A. *Ask whether there are family, friends, or clergy to call.*
The nurse should help the significant other identify support systems and resources that are helpful in coping with a crisis situation, such as the sudden death of a spouse.
B. *Inform the significant about the treatment the victim received.*
The significant other may be unable to process information during the crisis, and the nurse should focus on immediate needs for coping and support.
C. *Provide education about the stages of grief and loss.*
Educating the significant other about grief and loss is not an immediate priority in a crisis and should be provided after they begin to cope with the situation.
D. *Assess the significant other's level of anxiety.*
Although the nurse should assess the significant other for anxiety, the immediate intervention should include a directive approach to assist the spouse in dealing with the stressful event.

26. **The nurse is planning to lead a seminar for community health nurses on violence against women during pregnancy. Which statement describes an appropriate technique for assessing for violence?**
Rationales:
A. *Women should be assessed only if they are part of high-risk groups.*

Violence against women occurs in all ethnic groups and at all income levels.

B. ***Women may be assessed in the presence of young children but not intimate partners.***
It is important to assess women without their partners present; it is also important that verbal children not be present because they may repeat what is heard. Infants may be present.

C. ***The assessment only needs to be completed at the beginning of the pregnancy.***
Many women do not reveal violence the first time they are asked. As trust develops between the nurse and the client, the woman may be more comfortable sharing her story. Also, violence may start later in the pregnancy.

D. ***Women should be reassessed face-to-face by a nurse as the pregnancy progresses.***
More than one face-to-face interview elicits the highest reports of violence during pregnancy.

27. **The charge nurse reminds clients on the mental health unit that breakfast is at 8 AM, medications are given at 9 AM, and group therapy sessions begin at 10 AM. Which treatment modality has been implemented?**
Rationales:
A. ***Milieu therapy.***
Milieu therapy uses resources and activities in the environment to assist with improving social functioning and activities of daily living.

B. ***Behavior modification.***
Behavior modification involves changing behaviors using positive and negative reinforcements to allow desired activities or remove privileges.

C. ***Peer therapy***
Peer therapy is not a single therapeutic modality; it involves the interaction of peers who are responsible for supporting, sharing, and compromising within their peer group and milieu.

D. ***Problem-solving.***
Problem-solving is used in crisis intervention; it focuses on problem identification and ways to return to previous levels of functioning.

28. **The nurse is accompanying a male client to the radiography department when he becomes panic stricken at the elevator and states, "I can't get on that elevator." Which action should the nurse take first?**
Rationales:
A. ***Ask one more staff member to ride the elevator.***
One more staff member will not be able to mobilize the client to ride the elevator. The client must first recognize his feelings about the phobia and accept the need to change his behavior. Additional individuals in the elevator may actually increase the client's anxiety.

B. ***Offer a prescribed antianxiety medication.***

Offering an antianxiety medication may be needed to proceed with desensitization, but it not the first action.

C. ***Begin desensitization about riding the elevator.***
Desensitizing the client may be implemented, but first the client should identify his fears and recognize his anxiety.

D. ***Affirm the client's fears about riding the elevator.***
The nurse should first validate and allow the client to affirm his anxiety and fears about riding the elevator. Then options to initiate desensitization may be considered.

29. **A male client suffering from posttraumatic stress disorder (PTSD) is found one night trying to strangle his roommate. Which intervention is the nurse's highest priority?**
Rationales:
A. ***Give the client a sedative or hypnotic.***
While this may help the client with anxiety, safety is the priority.

B. ***Administer an antipsychotic medication.***
An antipsychotic medication is indicated if the client is psychotic and agitated; however, the nurse should ensure the safety of both clients first.

C. ***Assign a UAP to sit with the client.***
The nurse should implement safety precautions immediately and place a sitter with the patient.

D. ***Process with both clients about the event.***
Although both clients should talk about the incident, this is not an opportune time, and the clients should be separated to provide a safe environment.

30. **The nurse is updating the plan of care for a client who has a borderline personality disorder. Which intervention is most important to implement?**
Rationales:
A. ***Assign the same nurse to care for the client.***
The best intervention is to provide consistency and avoid splitting the staff by assigning the client to only one nurse.

B. ***Avoid challenging inappropriate behavior.***
The nurse should assist the client to recognize manipulative behavior and set limits on manipulative behaviors as necessary.

C. ***Limit the client's contact with other clients.***
Socialization should be encouraged to improve the client's social skills.

D. ***Remove consequences for acting-out behavior.***
Firm limits with clear expectations and consequences are needed for manipulative clients.

31. **A female adolescent is admitted to the mental health unit for anorexia nervosa. In planning care, what is the nurse's priority intervention?**
Rationales:

A. *Teach the client the importance of self-expression.*
Self-expression of feelings is important, but reestablishing normal eating habits and physiological integrity is the priority intervention.

B. *Supervise the client's activities during the day.*
The nurse should monitor and supervise the client's activities to prevent binging, purging, or avoiding meals.

C. *Include the client in daily group therapy.*
The client should be included in daily groups, but the priority is physiological needs and monitoring meals.

D. *Facilitate social interactions with others.*
The client should be given opportunities to socialize, but monitoring activities during the day, especially meals, is the priority.

32. **The charge nurse is planning the daily schedule for clients on the mental health unit. A male client who is manic should be assigned to which activity?**
Rationales:

A. *A basketball game in the gym.*
The client should avoid any potentially competitive physical activity, especially contact sports, that can stimulate aggressive acting out.

B. *Jogging at least 1 mile.*
Jogging is the best activity for this client because it is a noncompetitive physical activity, and it requires the use of large muscle groups that expend energy associated with mania.

C. *A table tennis game with a peer.*
The client should not be assigned to any competitive activities that can frustrate him and stimulate mood swings.

D. *Group therapy with the art therapist.*
A manic client may become disruptive and distracted in an art group; physical activity using large muscle groups is more effective in expending energy.

Leadership and Delegation

33. **A nurse is planning the client assignments for the night shift. The nursing team includes a registered nurse, a licensed practical nurse, and two unlicensed assistive personnel (UAP). Which duties should be delegated to the UAPs? (Select all that apply.)**
Rationales:

A. *Transport a client to the radiology department for a computed tomography (CT) scan.*

B. *Bathe a client with sickle cell disease who has multiple IV lines and a patient-controlled analgesia pump.*

C. *Turn a 92-year-old client who has end-stage heart failure and a do-not-resuscitate order.*

D. *Report to the healthcare provider the fingerstick blood glucose level of 2.72 mmol/L (49 mg/dL)*

E. *Feed a female client her first meal after she experienced a stroke.*
The UAP can perform noninvasive and nonsterile activities (options A, B, and C).

34. **A hospitalized client has been newly diagnosed with type 2 diabetes. Which task(s) can the RN delegate to the UAP? (Select all that apply.)**
Rationales:

A. *Contacting the dietitian for a prescribed consult.*

B. *Reviewing the client's insulin injection technique.*

C. *Obtaining the fingerstick blood glucose level before each meal and at bedtime.*

D. *Reminding the client to dry their toes carefully after a shower.*

E. *Talking to the client about foods that raise the blood glucose level.*
The UAP can collect and report data such as vital signs, height and weight, and capillary blood sugar results (C); perform hygiene tasks (D); and carry out clerical duties (A). Clients who need education or reinforcement of education require intervention by the RN or PN (B and E).

35. **The home health nurse evaluates the insulin preparation and administration technique of a 36-year-old male client newly diagnosed with diabetes. The client has been prescribed lispro insulin before each meal and glargine insulin once daily in the morning. Which finding indicates that the client needs further education?**
Rationales:

A. *He mixes glargine and lispro in the same syringe for the morning doses.*
Glargine and lispro must not be mixed with any other insulin.

B. *He leaves the insulin syringe in place for 10 seconds after injection.*
This ensures that all of the insulin is absorbed.

C. *He stores the opened insulin vials at room temperature in the cabinet.*
Insulin is stored at room temperature, out of direct sunlight.

D. *He recaps and disposes of the single-use insulin syringe.*
Clients may recap needles, but healthcare providers may not to reduce the risk of needlestick injury.

36. **At change of shift, the charge nurse assigns the UAP four clients. The RN should direct the UAP to take vital signs on which client first?**
Rationales:

A. *The 89-year-old with chronic obstructive pulmonary disease who is resting quietly on 2 L of oxygen and who needs assistance with a bath.*
This client is stable.

B. *The client who returned from surgery about 15 minutes ago and is requesting something to drink.*
This client has a set of time-sensitive vital signs, so this is a priority.

C. *The client newly diagnosed with type 2 diabetes who had a fingerstick blood glucose level of 5.0 mmol/L (90 mg/dL) and who needs help with breakfast.*
This client is stable.

D. *The newly admitted client with rheumatoid arthritis who needs to have hand splints reapplied to both hands.*
This client is stable.

37. **The arrythmia alarm sounds on a client on the telemetry unit, indicating that the client is in ventricular tachycardia. Place the nurse's actions for this client in order of priority from first to last.**
   Rationales:
   A. *Call the rapid response team.*
   B. *Assess for blood pressure.*
   C. *Give oxygen via nasal cannula.*
   D. *Bring defibrillator/crash cart to bedside.*
   E. *Document the incident.*
   Correct order: B, A, C, D, E. The nurse needs to first assess the client before calling the rapid response team. Also, if the patient is truly in ventricular tachycardia, it needs to be determined if it is pulseless v-tach or if the client has a pulse and blood pressure. If there is a pulse, the second action would be to call the rapid response team so that additional help is available. Then, the patient needs to have oxygen to maximize oxygenation of the circulating blood. The defibrillator needs to be brought to the bedside to be used for the cardioversion. The final activity is to document the findings.

38. **The nurse is reviewing the laboratory values of her assigned clients. Which client has an abnormal laboratory report that the nurse should communicate immediately to the healthcare provider?**
   Rationales:
   A. *The client who is postsplenectomy after a motor vehicle accident and has a hemoglobin of 109 mmol/L (10.9 g/dL).*
   This hemoglobin level is low but not at a critical level. This is not the priority.

B. *The client receiving warfarin (Coumadin) who has an international normalized ratio (INR) of 2.3.*
This lab value is therapeutic and expected.

C. *The 38-year-old client who is 24 hours postthyroidectomy and has a total calcium level of 2.35 mmol/L (9.4 mg/dL).*
This lab value is within normal limits.

D. *The newly admitted client with bipolar disorder with a lithium level of 2.5 mEq/L.*
Severe lithium toxicity occurs at 2.0 mEq/L; the nurse should notify the healthcare provider immediately.

39. **The nurse receives a change-of-shift report on her four acute care clients. Which action should the nurse take first?**
   Rationales:
   A. *Administer an antiemetic to a postoperative client who has been nauseated and is now vomiting.*
   Postoperative nausea and vomiting (PONV) are among the most common reactions after surgery. PONV can stress and irritate abdominal and gastrointestinal wounds, increase intracranial pressure in patients who had head and neck surgery, elevate intraocular pressure in patients who had eye surgery, and increase the risk for aspiration. Obtaining a prescription for relieving PONV will decrease these risks.

B. *Notify a family member of a client's impending transfer to the intensive care unit for angina and ST-segment changes.*
This is a change in status and should be performed after managing the PONV.

C. *Inform the healthcare provider of a potassium level of 5.2 mmol/L (mEq/L) in the client with end-stage renal disease.*
This is an expected finding in end-stage renal disease.

D. *Begin assessment rounds, starting with the palliative care client having a diagnosis of congestive failure.*
Assessing the client receiving palliative care is important; however, managing the client with PONV is the priority.

40. **The emergency department staff nurse is assigned four clients. Which client should the nurse assess first?**
   Rationales:
   A. *A preschooler with a barking cough, an O$_2$ saturation of 93% on room air, and occasional inspiratory stridor.*
   This is not a medical emergency. With an O$_2$ saturation of 93%, the child is not in acute respiratory distress.

B. *A 10-month-old with a tympanic temperature of 38.9°C (102°F) and green nasal drainage and who is pulling at her ears.*
The child has an infection and probably needs antibiotics, but this is not a medical emergency.

C. *A crying 8-month-old with a harsh, paroxysmal cough; an audible expiratory wheeze; and mild retractions.*
These symptoms are often seen with children with croup. While the child does need humidified air, they are not in acute respiratory distress.

D. *A clingy 3-year-old who has a sore throat and drooling and whose tongue slightly protrudes from his mouth*
Drooling, a history of sore throat, and a protruding tongue are classic manifestations of epiglottitis; this is a medical emergency. The throat can quickly occlude and cause respiratory arrest.

41. **The outpatient clinic nurse is reviewing phone messages from the previous night. Which client should the nurse call back first?**
Rationales:

A. *A woman at 30 weeks' gestation who has been diagnosed with mild preeclampsia who was unable to relieve her heartburn.*
A sign of a potential complication of eclampsia is epigastric pain, which may be indicative of liver damage and HELLP (hemolysis, elevated liver enzymes, low platelet count) syndrome, a medical emergency.

B. *A woman at 24 weeks' gestation who was crying about painful vulvar lesions and urinary frequency for the past 8 hours.*
This are concerns, possibly indications of a sexually transmitted disease. But these concerns do not take priority over the client with possible HELLP syndrome.

C. *A woman at 12 weeks' gestation who was recently discharged from the hospital with hyperemesis gravidarum and had had two episodes of vomiting in 6 hours.*
This client does need to be followed up with for possible dehydration, but the client with possible HELLP syndrome takes precedence.

D. *A woman with type 1 diabetes who tested positive with a home pregnancy kit and was worried about managing her diabetes.*
This client needs education, but this is not a priority.

42. **The clinic nurse suspects that a 2-year-old child is being abused. Which assessment finding(s) would support this? (Select all that apply.)**
Rationales:

A. *Petechiae in a straight line on the chest.*
Petechiae on the chest may be the result of the coining procedure, a cultural practice among Southeast Asian populations.

B. *Gray-blue pigmented areas on the sacral region.*

These are Mongolian spots, blue areas commonly located on the sacral region that are consistent in shape and color.

C. ***Bald patches on the scalp.***
Bald patches typically are symmetrical and are indicative of physical abuse.

D. *Ear tugging and crying.*
Ear tugging and crying are typical signs of otitis media.

E. ***Symmetrical burns on the hands.***
Symmetrical burns are indicative of physical abuse.

43. **The nurse is caring for a client who had a thoracotomy 48 hours ago and now has left lower lobe chest tubes. The nurse notes that a chest tube is not tidaling. Which action should the nurse take first?**
Rationales:

A. ***Check for kinks in the chest drainage system.***
Normal fluctuation of the water, called tidaling, reflects the intrapleural pressure during inspiration and expiration. If no tidaling is observed (rising with inspiration and falling with expiration in a spontaneously breathing patient), the drainage system may be blocked. An absence of fluctuation may mean that the lung has fully healed (which is unlikely at 48 hours), or it can mean that there is an obstruction in the chest tube. A simple step is to ensure that there are no kinks that would occlude the chest tube and prevent lung drainage and expansion.

B. *Assess the heart rate and blood pressure.*
Checking the heart rate and blood pressure is not directly related to the lack of chest tube drainage.

C. *Notify the rapid response team immediately.*
Although the nurse should immediately notify the rapid response team for tracheal deviation, sudden onset of dyspnea, or mediastinal shift, the absence of tidaling may not be a medical emergency.

D. *Reconnect the chest tube to wall suction.*
When a chest tube is connected to wall suction, tidaling may stop. The nurse should disconnect the tube, not reconnect it, to observe for tidaling.

44. **While the nurse is caring for a client who has had a myocardial infarction, the monitor alarm sounds, and the nurse notes ventricular fibrillation. What is the nurse's first course of action?**
Rationales:

A. *Notify the healthcare provider.*
This may be an appropriate action after assessment of the client's clinical status.

B. *Increase the oxygen concentration.*
This may be an appropriate action after assessment of the client's clinical status.

C. *Assess the client.*
   If a monitor alarm sounds, the nurse should first assess the client's clinical status to see whether the problem is an actual dysrhythmia or a monitoring system malfunction.
D. *Prepare to defibrillate the client.*
   This may be an appropriate action after assessment of the client's clinical status.

45. **The healthcare provider has prescribed the removal of a client's internal jugular central line catheter. To remove the catheter safely, the nurse should give which intervention(s) the highest priority? (Select all that apply.)**
   Rationales:
   A. *Carefully remove the bio-occlusive dressing.*
      Removing the bio-occlusive dressing is important, but it is not a safety priority.
   B. *Place the client in the Trendelenburg position.*
      The procedure for removing the catheter safely is: (1) place the client in the Trendelenburg position, (2) have the client take a deep breath and hold it, and (3) gently withdraw the catheter while applying direct pressure with sterile gauze. Holding the breath creates positive pressure in the intrathoracic space, and the Trendelenburg position minimizes the risk of air entering the catheter.
   C. *Send the catheter tip to the lab for culture and sensitivity.*
      The catheter tip may or may not be sent to the lab, depending on the protocol of the facility.
   D. *Have the client hold a deep breath during removal.*
      See the explanation for B.
   E. *Apply pressure for 20 minutes after removal of the catheter.*
      Applying pressure for 20 minutes is a technique used in arterial line withdrawal to prevent bleeding.

46. **The nurse who usually works on the orthopedic surgery unit is floating to a cardiovascular unit. Which client would be best to assign to the float nurse?**
   Rationales:
   A. *Client scheduled for a heart catheterization this morning.*
      Preparing the client for a cardiac catheterization requires specialized information, and it would be best to assign to the nurse who usually works on the cardiovascular unit.
   B. *Client admitted last night for chest pain.*
      This client requires close monitoring by the nurse who has additional education about cardiac issues.
   C. *Client who underwent popliteal bypass surgery yesterday.*
      This would require similar care to a client who had just had lower extremity orthopedic surgery and would be the safest assignment for this nurse.

D. *Client who has heart failure and is scheduled for a stress test today.*
   Preparing the client for a stress test requires specialized information and would be best to assign to the nurse who usually works on the cardiovascular unit.

47. **The nurse is admitting a client who is a paraplegic and has a nonhealing pressure injury with a possible methicillin-resistant Staphylococcus aureus infection. A UAP and PN are assigned to the RN's team. Which tasks should be delegated to the PN? (Select all that apply.)**
   Rationales:
   A. *Place the client in isolation.*
      This task can be safely assigned to the UAP.
   B. *Complete a dressing change.*
      This task is within the scope of practice for the PN.
   C. *Assess and document the wound.*
      Initial assessment of a wound should be completed by the registered nurse.
   D. *Insert a urinary catheter.*
      This task is within the scope of practice for the PN.
   E. *Administer oral pain medications.*
      This task is within the scope of practice for the PN.

48. **The nursing supervisor calls the nurse on a step-down unit about the need for a bed for an unstable patient from the medical unit. Which client should the nurse transfer to the medical unit in order to receive this unstable client?**
   Rationales:
   A. *A client admitted for an ST-elevation myocardial infarction (STEMI) who just returned from having a cardiac catheterization performed.*
      This patient needs close monitoring for the first 24 hours and should remain on the step-down unit.
   B. *A client diagnosed with congestive heart failure who is receiving IV infusion of furosemide.*
      This patient could be safely taken care of on a medical-surgical unit.
   C. *A client with possible Guillain-Barré syndrome who may need an exchange transfusion.*
      This patient needs close monitoring and should remain in the step-down unit.
   D. *A client in hypertensive crisis who is on a sodium nitroprusside drip.*
      Patients on a nitroprusside drip need frequent vital signs and close monitoring. This patient should remain on the step-down unit.

49. **When accessing the medication dispensing system (Pyxis), the nurse finds chlorpropamide in the drawer instead of the expected chlorpromazine.**

Which actions should the nurse take? (Select all that apply.)

Rationales:
A. *Remove the tablets of chlorpropamide.*
B. *Notify the pharmacy about the mistake.*
C. *Place an incident or occurrence report.*
D. *Be extra vigilant because the pharmacy is making mistakes.*
E. *Place a warning note on the Pyxis machine.*
   The nurse needs to ensure that others do not give the wrong medication, so the tablets of chlorpropamide need to be removed and returned to the pharmacy (A). The pharmacy needs to be made aware of the error (B) and an incident (also called an occurrence) report completed (C) to help prevent the error in the future. The other options (E and D) are not needed at this time.

50. The nurse is calling the healthcare provider (HCP) about a client's current needs. What is the best way to communicate?

Rationales:
A. *Call the HCP with the request and a recommendation.*
   Letting the physician know the needs of the patient is important, but key information may be missed using this way to communicate.
B. *Use the SBAR (situation, background, assessment, recommendation) tool regardless for communication.*
   Using the SBAR format ensures that all key information is given and is the best way to communicate.
C. *Send a text message or page with the needed order.*
   This may be an ineffective way to communicate and may not ensure that all key information is given. Additionally, if both phones are not encrypted, this may place the patient's information at risk.
D. *Ask the HCP to come back to the unit to discuss the client's needs.*
   Although face-to-face communication is often valuable, this does not ensure that all key information is communicated.

51. The healthcare provider plans to do a paracentesis on a client with cirrhosis in 1 hour. In what order should the nurse perform the following activities?

Rationales:
A. *Ensure that the informed consent has been obtained.*
B. *Measure the client's abdominal girth.*
C. *Have the patient empty his or her bladder.*
D. *Assemble needed equipment.*
E. *Administer oral pain medication.*

Rationales:
   Correct order: A, E, C, B, D

Before a procedure can be completed, it is essential to have an informed consent (A). Oral pain medication can then be given (after the consent has been obtained) to help the patient relax during the procedure (E). The client then needs to empty his or her bladder before the procedure to prevent accidentally puncturing the bladder (C). After the bladder is empty, a baseline abdominal girth is obtained (B). Finally, the nurse needs to assemble the correct equipment for the procedure (D).

52. The nurse receives report on a client from the emergency department with a diagnosis of pneumonia. Which intervention has the highest priority?

Rationales:
A. *Obtain blood cultures.*
   Blood cultures are not needed unless the client is suspected of being septic.
B. *Initiate prescribed antibiotics.*
   Studies have shown that the sooner antibiotics are started, the better the outcomes. Current requirements include antibiotic administration within 2 hours of diagnosis. This is the priority.
C. *Place the client in isolation.*
   The question does not state what organism is causing the pneumonia, so this may not be needed.
D. *Obtain an accurate weight.*
   This would be needed if the antibiotic is weight based but is not usually a priority.

53. The nurse is part of the triage team at a disaster. Which client should be seen first?

Rationales:
A. *A 90-year-old woman with a crushed pelvis and head injuries.*
   This client would be triaged black.
B. *A 21-year-old male screaming in pain from a broken leg.*
   This client's injuries are not life-threatening, and he can wait to be seen.
C. *A 30-year-old woman with a flail chest secondary to a puncture wound to the chest.*
   The flail chest causes the heart to become unstable and is life-threatening. This client needs to be seen immediately.
D. *A 12-year-old crying with multiple lacerations to the legs.*
   Although the child needs to be comforted, the injuries are not life-threatening, and this client can wait for treatment.

54. The triage nurse in the emergency room is assessing four clients. Which client requires the most immediate intervention?

Rationales:

A. ***The client who arrived via ambulance with numbness and tingling of his left arm and face.***
The client may be experiencing a stroke and requires immediate assessment and interventions. If interventions are initiated quickly, the complications may be mitigated.

B. **The adult client who had a seizure at home who is sleeping on his left side.**
While a seizure is highly concerning, the priority is the client who may be diagnosed with a stroke.

C. **The 60-year-old client who complains of frequent urination and has a blood sugar of 16.7 mmol/L (300 mg/dL).**
An elevated blood sugar may indicate diabetes, and polyuria is an expected symptom. It is considered urgent and not emergent.

D. **The middle-aged client who presents with severe unilateral back pain and previous history of kidney stones.**
Although this is highly concerning, the client exhibiting symptoms of a stroke is a higher priority.

55. **After the change-of-shift report on an orthopedic floor, which client should the nurse assess first?**
Rationales:

A. *A client who had surgery yesterday and has a temperature of 37.6°C (99.7°F).*
A slight increase in temperature is expected postoperatively.

B. ***A client who is complaining of numbness and tingling distal to the fracture site.***
This is a sign of compartment syndrome. This client needs to be assessed first.

C. *A client who had a left leg amputation and states he is experiencing pain in the left foot.*
Phantom pain is expected after an amputation and should be treated but is not as critical as assessing for compartment syndrome.

D. *A client who is extremely upset with their care and is requesting to speak with the manager.*
This is a customer service issue and needs to be addressed but is not a high priority.

56. **The nurse is administering medications to a client admitted for an overdose and a history of substance abuse. Which intervention(s) are priorities to include in this client's plan of care? (Select all that apply.)**
Rationales:

A. *Allow the client to take medications independently.*
With a history of substance abuse, the nurse needs to observe the client as medications are taken.

B. ***Ensure that all medications have been swallowed before leaving the client's room.***
To ensure that medications are not being hoarded or kept to be taken at a later time, the nurse needs to watch the client swallow his or her medications.

C. ***Request that oral pain medications be changed from tablet to oral suspension.***
Liquid forms of medications are harder to save to be taken later so are often used for clients with a history of substance abuse.

D. *Give flumazenil every 6 hours around the clock.*
Flumazenil is used to reverse benzodiazepine overdose and is given as needed, not around the clock.

E. *Only give medications to the client via the intravenous route.*
There is no indication to give medications intravenously.

57. **The nurse is returning phone calls to clients who are cared for at an outpatient mental health center. Which client should the nurse call first?**
Rationales:

A. ***The young mother diagnosed with schizophrenia who is hearing voices say that they are pursuing her children.***
This client is at risk for hurting herself or her children. She needs to be seen first.

B. *The elderly male at an assisted living facility who says he wants to end it all.*
This client is at risk for committing suicide, but he lives in a facility where there is staff that the nurse can notify about his thoughts. The staff can stay with him until he can be brought into the clinic.

C. *The female client diagnosed with bipolar disorder who is manic and has not slept for 48 hours.*
Although this client needs to be seen to have her medications adjusted, she is not the priority client.

D. *The teenager diagnosed with bulimia whose mother called and reported that she found her daughter purging.*
This client does need to be seen but is not in imminent danger.

58. **An 18-year-old female is being discharged after delivering a healthy baby. She has a cousin whose baby died from sudden infant death syndrome (SIDS). The client seems to know many of the precautions to take. Which information does the nurse need to correct?**
Rationales:

A. *Always place infants on their backs to sleep.*
This is correct. Babies should be placed on their backs.

B. *Room sharing has been shown to decrease SIDS.*
This is correct. Studies show that room sharing does decrease SIDS.

C. *Keep the crib free of stuffed animals and crib pads.*

This is correct. The bed should be free of items that could cause suffocation.

D. ***Sleeping with the baby can alert the mother to changes.***

Sleeping with the baby increases the risk for injury and SIDS for infants.

59. **A 4-year-old admitted with pneumonia weighs 18 kg. The healthcare provider has prescribed vancomycin 40 mg/kg/day IV. The order states to divide the dose and give it three times daily. How many mg of vancomycin should the child receive in each dose? (Round the answer to the nearest whole number.)**

_____ mg/dose

Rationales:

$$18\ mg \times \frac{40\ mg}{kg} = \frac{720\ mg}{kg}$$

$$\frac{720\ mg}{3} = \frac{240\ mg}{dose}$$

60. **The nurse needs to initiate an IV on an 8-year-old child. Which intervention(s) is/are appropriate? (Select all that apply).**

Rationales:

A. ***Start the IV in the treatment room, not the child's room.***

The child's room is a safe zone, and painful treatments should not be performed in the child's room.

B. *Apply a lidocaine-based cream for a few minutes before starting the IV.*

To be effective, the cream needs to be applied for about 1 hour before the IV is started.

C. *Ask the parents to leave the room while performing the procedure.*

Having parents present can help the child cope with this procedure.

D. ***Encourage the child to use guided imagery to cope.***

Children at this age can understand and participate in guided imagery.

E. *Offer the child a reward if they cooperate during the procedure.*

Offering the child a reward does not help the child to cope with the IV insertion.

Notes